EVIDENCE BASED MEDICINE – CLOSER TO PATIENTS OR SCIENTISTS?

Edited by **Nikolaos M. Sitaras**

Evidence Based Medicine – Closer to Patients or Scientists?
Edited by Nikolaos M. Sitaras

Published by InTech

Janeza Trdine 9, 51000 Rijeka, Croatia

Publishing Process Manager Martina Blecic

Technical Editor Teodora Smiljanic

Cover Designer InTech Design Team

Additional hard copies can be obtained from orders@intechopen.com

Evidence Based Medicine – Closer to Patients or Scientists?, Edited by Nikolaos M. Sitaras
p. cm.
ISBN 978-953-51-0504-6

For EU product safety concerns:
IN TECH d.o.o., Prolaz Marije Krucifikse Kozulić 3, 51000 Rijeka, Croatia,
info@intechopen.com or visit our website at intechopen.com.

Meet the editor

Dr Nikolaos M. Sitaras, MD, PhD, is an Associate Professor of Pharmacology, Department of Pharmacology, Medical School, University of Athens, Athens, Greece.

Contents

Preface

Evidence-based, in general, is the term that characterizes many decision making processes in modern society and science. From justice to politics. To medicine.

Evidence-based medicine (EBM) was introduced to the best benefit of the patient. It has transformed the *pathophysiological approach* to the *outcome approach* of today's treatments. *Disease- oriented* to *patient- oriented* medicine. And, for some, daily medical practice from *patient oriented* to *case oriented* medicine. Evidence has changed the paternalistic way of medical practice. And gave room to patients, who show a tendency towards partnership.

The only certain in medical science is uncertainty. Therefore, medicine relies more and more to statistics. But the significant does not always dignify the essential. As William Osler quoted, "if it was not for differences among individuals, the Art of Medicine could be Science in addition".

Statistical significance is not enough. Importance is hidden under the clinical influence of evidence. And according to Gertrude Stein, "for a difference to be different it must make a difference".

Although EBM has introduced a different way of thinking in the day to day medical practice, there is plenty of space for implementation and improvement. And the dispute remains: should "Evidence-based Medicine" be the new "Faith-based Medicine"?

Dr Nikolaos M. Sitaras
Athens University, Medical School,
Department of Experimental Pharmacology,
Athens,
Greece

1

Designing, Conducting and Reporting Randomised Controlled Trials: A Few Key Points

Hamidreza Mahboobi[1], Tahereh Khorgoei[2] and Neha Bansal[3]
[1]*Hormozgan University of Medical Sciences, Student Research Committee,*
[2]*Hormozgan University of Medical Sciences, Infectious and Tropical Disease Research Center,*
[3]*Seth G.S. Medical College,*
[1,2]*Iran*
[3]*India*

1. Introduction

Randomized Controlled Trials (RCTs) are the most valuable study which play an important role in the field of medicine. Other study types including descriptive studies (e.g. case reports, case series, cross-sectional studies) and certain analytical studies (e.g. case control studies, cohort studies) are also important pieces of evidence but RCTs which are designed for evaluation of the interventions in clinical practice are probably the highest level of evidence in the pyramid of Evidence Based Medicine. It is simple, yet the most powerful tool in modern clinical research.

2. RCTs: Top of the evidence-pyramid

RCTs are considered the most powerful evidence that exists. This is most probably due to the fact that 'randomizing' people into two different groups probably takes care of all the confounding factors and equals out all the causes which may affect the final result of the study.

This is mostly because of their accurate design. This reduces any possibility of bias in the result. Every year, the numbers of RCTs that are published in Medical Journals are increasing and thus, they have a great effect on changing the way medical science is practiced all over the world. Evidence-Based Medicine is highly dependent on the RCTs.

Therefore designing, conducting and reporting RCTs is an important aspect of medical science and all medical professionals should learn these skills. Critical appraisal of RCTs is probably as important as conducting them. All medical professionals need to understand and evaluate RCTs for the possibility of bias or any shortcomings. RCT results translate directly into changing clinical practice. Hence, it is important that they are free of bias and are strong in their design and execution.

3. RCTs: The other side of the coin

However, RCTs are not far from their fair share of disadvantages. They may be the most powerful tool in the world of research but many ethical and practical concerns limit their use.

3.1. Not all randomized trials are unethical. However, a RCT may be ethical but infeasible. This may be due to difficulties in randomization or recruitment. For example, interventions like cancer screening at an early age might have an extremely long follow up with not may positive outcomes.

3.2. Once a convention is set in the community or a particular intervention gains popularity, it is tough convincing the subjects to "experiment" with their alternative options. A recent attempt to conduct a trial of counselling in general practice failed when practitioners declined to recruit patients to be allocated at random.

3.3. Certain populations of people may have certain strong ideologies and preferences. This may also limit recruitment and result in bias outcomes if not accounted for and accommodated within the study design.

3.4. Randomised trials are not always practical for evaluation of rare diseases or rare outcomes or even outcomes which take a long time to develop.

3.5. A successful and valid RCT requires a large sample size because the outcomes generally have smaller effects and a large measurable difference is required when comparing two groups of interventions. So, the larger the sample size, the better the randomized trial but the larger the financial constraints as well as the time required for the trial to be completed.

3.6. They also have a fairly large drop-out rates and a huge population of the sample size is often lost to follow up making it even harder to assess the final results.

3.7. Even with the people who do follow up, not all religiously adhere to the regimen prescribed to them and some may even be totally non-compliant.

3.8. Since they require a lot of time and manpower, they are fairly expensive to conduct. Financial constraints are probably the most common reason for a trial to be shelved.

3.9. Randomized trials have a huge ethical dilemma. If an intervention is considered inferior to the current treatment modality, exposing some patients to it and not others (or exposing one group to placebo and the other to the treatment) is often thought unethical. For example, a non-random study suggested that multivitamin supplementation during pregnancy could prevent neural tube defects in children. Even though the study was seriously flawed, ethics committees were unwilling to deprive patients of this potentially useful treatment, making it difficult to carry out the trial which later showed that folic acid was the effective part of the multivitamin cocktail.

Thus, these randomized trials should only be undertaken if there is an important question which needs to be answered by the physician and other small scale observational or analytical studies justify its conduction.

4. Justification of your trial: Ask two keys questions

A simple way of knowing if you should go through the trouble of conducting the randomized trial is to ask yourself these two simple questions:

4.1. Is the intervention well enough developed to permit evaluation?

This can be especially difficult to decide when new interventions are heavily dependent on clinicians' skills (surgical procedures[7] or "talk" therapies).

4.2. Is there preliminary evidence that the intervention is likely to be beneficial (from observational studies), including some appreciation of the size of the likely treatment effect?

Such information is needed to estimate sample sizes and justify the expense of a trial.

However, there is another side of the story. Failure to perform these important trials which should have been conducted may sometimes result in harmful treatments being used continuously without validation and evaluation. For example, neonates were widely treated with high concentrations of oxygen until randomized trials identified oxygen as a risk factor for retinopathy of prematurity.

Other study designs, including non-randomised controlled trials, can detect associations between an intervention and an outcome. But they cannot rule out the possibility that the association was caused by a third factor linked to both intervention and outcome. Double blinding ensures that the preconceived views of subjects and clinicians cannot systematically bias the assessment of outcomes.

5. History of randomised controlled trials

Daniel Judah has been thought to have conducted the first and earliest recorded clinical trial which dates back to approximately 600 B.C. He compared the health effects of the vegetarian diet with those of a royal Babylonian diet over a 10-day period. The trial was obviously not even close to the current modern standards set for trials and was majorly flawed with allocation bias, ascertainment bias, and confounding by divine intervention, but the report has influenced medical decision for now over two millennia.

The 19th century saw a steep development curve in the history of clinical trials. In 1836, the editor of the *American Journal of Medical Sciences* wrote an introduction to an article that he considered "one of the most important medical works of the present century, marking the start of a new era of science," and stated that the article was "the first formal exposition of the results of the only true method of investigation in regard to the therapeutic value of remedial agents." This article was the French study on bloodletting in treatment of pneumonia by P. C. A. Louis. Sir Austin Bradford Hill takes all the credit for the modern concepts of randomization trials. The Medical Research Council trials on streptomycin for pulmonary tuberculosis are rightly regarded as a landmark that ushered in a new era of medicine. Since Hill's pioneering achievement, the methodology of the randomized controlled trial has been increasingly accepted and the number of randomized controlled trials reported has grown exponentially. The Cochrane Library already lists more than 150,000 such trials, and they have become the underlying basis for what is currently called "evidence-based medicine"

6. Evidence supporting randomised trials

Enough evidence exists that a successful RCT is one which is well-designed. These RCTs are superior to other study designs in estimating an intervention's true effect. Meta-analysis of controlled trials shows that failure to conceal random allocation and the absence of double blinding yield exaggerated estimates of treatment effects.

It is also well known that well-matched comparison-group designs may be a good alternative when an RCT is not feasible.

7. Issues in designing and conducting RCTs

As, mentioned before RCTs are conducted to evaluate the importance of an intervention of any sorts. They can be used to understand the effectiveness of a screening test or the effect of any surgical or medical intervention by comparing the outcomes like mortality or disease recurrence.

Let's discuss several important issues in designing and conducting of RCTs.

7.1 Inclusion and exclusion criteria

In all study types the researchers need to define their target population and the criteria for inclusion and exclusion of every individual in the study. This forms an important aspect of the trial which needs to be decided before starting the trial.

Accurate definition of the study population in RCTs is extremely important and some key pointers are:

7.1.1. In RCTs, the researcher needs to make an intervention on the study population and it is required that these candidates in the study are eligible for receiving the intervention according to the current guidelines.

7.1.2. If the intervention is contraindicated in a population, then that population meets the exclusion criteria of the study target.

7.1.3. Sometimes it is difficult to assess the effect of an intervention in a large population because that needs a large sample size. So the researcher intervenes on a specific portion of the population (for example a specific sex or age group).

7.1.4. Case selection bias is one of the most important bias in RCTs which can be prevented by using appropriate inclusion and exclusion criteria.

Sometimes, the same criteria can be used as either for inclusion or exclusion from the study. For example, a specific drug reaction can serve as both depending on what the researcher wants to study. It can be an inclusion criterion if the study is about a particular drug and the associated adverse reaction. It can also be an exclusion criterion in case the investigator wants to analyze the efficacy of the drug.

The researchers need to report the exact number of the individuals assessed intending to meet the inclusion criteria, the exact number of individuals included in the study after fulfilling all inclusion and exclusion criteria, the exact number of individuals excluded from the study at the end along with the reasons for the same. It is useful to note that unwillingness of an individual to receive the intervention is an exclusion criterion.

7.2 Study designs

All randomized trials usually have similar study design. However, still some differences exist. If classified according to the patient exposure and the response to the intervention, the following styles exist:

7.2.1 Parallel design

This is the most popular design and is based on the comparison of the effects of the intervention in the case group with the control group or another intervention group. The two groups receive a maximum of one intervention. Normally two parallel groups with equal sample size will be selected through a randomized selection. However, at times the number of the two groups isn't equal. It is important that the researcher reports this as well as the ratio of the individuals in the two groups at the time of reporting the trial.

Randomized trials can also be done by involving more than two groups. It is then known as a multi-arm parallel RCT.

7.2.2 Cross-over design

Each participant receives all the interventions involved in the trial. The sequential order in which they receive them is decided randomly. This study design however should be limited to stable chronic conditions where the disease profile doesn't fluctuate over time as well as short interventions. Also a key concern in these trials is the adequate washout period between the two therapies in order to avoid the carry-on effect.

7.2.3 Factorial design

This is a complex design where more answers can be found in a single trial. The two or more interventions are compared between themselves as well as a control group. Since RCTs are expensive to conduct, it's better that we get more answers in a single trial.

Due to such differences, it is important that the study design is described in detail at the time of reporting the trial. This helps the reader a much better understanding of the research conducted. All the study designs must be considered and the best one chosen at the time of designing one's RCT.

Usually the study design is fixed once the protocol is submitted and the researchers don't change it till end of the study. However, sometimes there is need to modify the study due to various reasons. It is important that researchers explain the cause of the same and also the outline the changes in the RCT design in detail.

7.3 Intervention

One of the most important issues in RCTs is the intervention. Researchers need to answer several questions about this aspect before even starting their trial.

An intervention can be a drug or device. It can be used for prevention or treatment. For drugs it is important to carefully determine the dosage, timing, duration and administration route. All information about the drug needs to be provided to the reader at the time of reporting. Even the manufacturer of the drug or device can be mentioned for the sake of complete reporting and easy reproducibility of the trial if required.

Even very small differences either in the type, dosage, duration or the route of administration may lead to a significant difference in the outcomes. The intervention should be obvious in order to give the possibility of comparison to other study to the researchers as well as a chance to reproduce the results if required.

7.4 Outcome/ Results

Probably the most important think we are looking for in a randomized trial article are the outcomes or the results. These can be divided into primary and secondary outcomes. They should have been determined before even starting the study.

Primary outcome is the main intervention outcome. Other study outcomes aer put in the category of secondary outcomes. For example the drug side effects are usually put in that category.

Another important issue in the outcomes is the 'measures' used to measure these outcomes. The outcomes may be laboratory test results. For these outcomes, it is important to list the methodology for the measurement, kits used for the same as well as the manufacturer where they are produced.

Other type of outcome is the clinical outcome. For this, it is important to mention the guidelines used by the researcher for the determination of the variable as well as the name of that person (e.g. General physician, specialists or medical students).

It is recommended that before selection of the primary and secondary outcomes the researchers reviews the literature thoroughly and chooses the similar outcomes in similar studies. This is important for comparing the results of the evidence already out there with their study.

An advantage of designing a trial with clearly pre-determined inclusion criteria/exclusion criteria, intervention and outcomes which are similar to other studies, is the possibility of collecting these data to form a meta-analysis which gives us even more clarity and consolidates all the evidence to give a final conclusion.

7.5 Sample size

A small sample size is unable to show all differences between case and control group. As we mentioned before, the effects are usually small and thus, we need to demonstrate large results to show sizable difference and this is why we need a large sample size. However, large sample sizes need more time and budget. There are also issues with recruitment and reaching out to large populations. Sample size should be determined after a thorough literature review and full access to previous studies in populations similar to the current study and also after determination of the power of the study. The sample size is the answer to the power of the study and simply answers the question: how many participants are needed in order to show the difference in a particular outcome in a certain statistical significance?

Sample size should be determined using sample size calculator software or the standard formula. It is recommended to consult a statistician for calculation of the study sample size.

7.6 Randomization

Randomization is what gives the RCTs its strength. In RCTs patients are randomly assigned into the two or more study groups and each individual has an equal chance to be assigned to any group. The clinician, the investigators or the patient have no choice in the allocation. This prevents the selection bias. Random allocation ensures no systematic differences between intervention groups in factors, known and unknown, that may affect outcome. No other study design allows this kind of a balance. It is crucial that the investigators pre define the allocation guidelines and stick by it till the end of the trial. It is extremely important that the guidelines are not modified at any point in the trial. Randomization can be done in several different methods.

The easiest method to do randomization of the sample is 'simple randomization'. In this method, individuals are assigned equally to the groups using a random process, for example, a computer generated list of random numbers. Other methods like blocked randomization and stratified randomization are more complex, less common and are usually used for very specific trials. Blocked randomization aims to numerical balance between groups and stratified randomization aims to balance characteristics between the groups.

7.7 Blinding

Blinding means that the person is not aware of what group he/she is in and what treatment or placebo he/she is receiving. According to the various levels of blinding like blinding the participants, researchers, outcome assessors and statisticians, RCTs are divided into four types: open label, single blinded, double blinded and triple blinded RCTs. Due to confusions and discrepancies about who exactly was blinded in the single and double and triple blinded studies, The 2010 CONSORT guidelines specify that authors should not use these terms. It is required to report the details of the blinding like "If done, who was blinded after assignment to interventions (for example, participants, care providers, those assessing outcomes) and how."

Blinding obviously helps to prevent personal bias in the study which is a huge concern in conducting a RCT. Every effort should be made to reduce any bias as much as possible. In case the study population is neonates, researchers may decide not to use blinding because of the differences in interventions like oral or IV feeds. The most prevalent type of blinding is the double blinded design where the investigator and the patient are both unaware of the details of who is in which group.

7.8 Statistical analysis

The most common statistical tests used for all type of papers are descriptive. These tests include mean and standard deviation for quantitative variables and frequency and percentage for qualitative variables. They also use Chi-square test or Exact fisher test for comparison and the T tests are also commonly used. Other descriptive statistical tests are less commonly used. However, researchers may need other statistical tests for subgroup analysis and adjusted analysis.

Two main ways to analyze RCTs are per protocol analysis and intent to treat analysis. In per protocol analysis, analysis will be done based on the groups which the patients are assigned into, but in intent to treat analysis the analysis is based on receiving treatment or not.

Some RCTs need large sample sizes and may continue for a long time. The researchers may decide to cease the study if significant difference was observed in important study outcomes. For example if a specific drug be associated with significant increase in a side effect, then the study should be stopped. Also if a significant improvement be observed during the study, the researchers can stop the study. To reach this aim interim analysis can be done. But the number of interim analysis, the time, the individuals who will do it and the conditions in which the study will stop should be clear.

8. Clinical trial registry

All RCTs need to be registered in international clinical trial registry databases before starting enrolment of study participants. Once the researchers register their clinical trial in a clinical trial registry database they will receive a unique trial registry number.

Almost all medical journals request their authors mention their trial registry number in the abstract of their paper. The editors of these journals avoid publication of RCTs without trial registry number even if they have high quality in study design and writing.

According to the registry database where the researchers register their clinical trial, detailed information about the trial is needed by them.

This information includes: Title, purpose, condition which the study is studying in detail, type, name and dosage and all other information about the intervention, study type, allocation, endpoints and outcomes, intervention model, masking (Blinding), the number of patient enrolled in the study, study start and completion dates, inclusion and exclusion criteria etc.

RCT registration has several benefits. They are a good source of previous trials and it is possible to search and reach the content of the registered RCTs easily.

During the registration the researchers needs to review all important issues in the study design and methodology of the research. This helps them to reduce bias in their design and consider all aspect of the RCT design.

All RCTs need to obtain the ethics approval of the committee of the institute or the hospital where they want to conduct the trial. This practice will guarantee that all the RCTs published in the top-notch high impact medical journals are validated and ethically correct.

The International Clinical Trial Registry Platform (ICTRP) has introduced ten primary registries in its registry network which can register the clinical trial with their profile and the link to their website

- Australasian New Zealand Clinical Trial Registry
- Brazilian Clinical Trial Registry
- Chinese Clinical Trial Registry
- Clinical Research Information Service (CRIS) , Republic of Korea
- Clinical Trial Registry - India
- Cuban Public Registry of Clinical Trials
- EU Clinical Trial Registry
- German Clinical Trial Registry
- Iranian Registry of Clinical Trials
- Japan Primary Registries Network

9. Summary

Randomised controlled trials are the most rigorous way of determining whether a cause-effect relation exists between treatment and outcome and for assessing the cost effectiveness of a treatment. Some key pointers at a glance are:

9.1. Random allocation to intervention groups

9.2. Patients and trialists should remain unaware of which treatment was given until the study is completed-although such double blind studies are not always feasible or appropriate

9.3. All intervention groups are treated identically except for the experimental treatment

9.4. Patients are normally analysed within the group to which they were allocated, irrespective of whether they experienced the intended intervention (intention to treat analysis)

9.5. The analysis is focused on estimating the size of the difference in predefined outcomes between intervention groups.

Given that poor design may lead to biased outcomes, investigators should strive for methodological rigour and report their work in enough detail for others to assess its quality.

10. References

Stolberg HO et al. Fundamentals of Clinical Research for Radiologists. AJR 2004;183:1539–1544.

Afshar Z, et al. Research Mentorship Program (RMP) to Enhance the Research Productivity in a Psychiatric Hospital: First Report. Electronic Physician. 2011;3(4):442-445.

Mahboobi H, et al. Current form of randomized controlled trials. Annals of Pediatric Cardiology. 2011;4(1):90.

Mahboobi H, et al. Designing a Research Mentorship Program (RMP) to enhance research productivity at Ebne-Sina psychiatric hospital. Australasian Medical Journal. 2010;1(2):180-2.

Mahboobi H, et al. Evidence-based medicine for medical students. Aust Med J. 2010;1:190-3.

Mahboobi H, et al. Have we something to replace evidence based medicine? Annals of Cardiac Anaesthesia. 2011;14(3):246.

Mahboobi H, et al. Mentorship in Medical Students researches. Electronic Physician 2011; 3(4):414-415.

Marcinkiewicz M et al. The Impact of the Internet on the Doctor-Patient Relationship. Australasian Medical Journal 2009; 2(5):1-6.

Schulz KF et al. CONSORT 2010 Statement: updated guidelines for reporting parallel group randomised trials. Ann Int Med 2010;152.

2

Innovating Medical Knowledge: Understanding Evidence-Based Medicine as a Socio-Medical Phenomenon

Maya J. Goldenberg
University of Guelph, Canada

1. Introduction

Because few would object to evidence-based medicine's (EBM) principal task of basing medical decisionmaking on the most judicious and up-to-date evidence, the debate over this prolific movement may seem puzzling. Who, one may ask, could be against evidence (Carr-Hill, 2006)? Yet this question belies the sophistication of the evidence-based movement. This chapter presents the evidence-based approach as a socio-medical phenomenon and seeks to explain and negotiate the points of disagreement between supporters and detractors. This is done by casting EBM as more than the simple application of research findings to clinical care and improved health outcomes, but rather an umbrella term that harnesses a specific set of pedagogical objectives (some rather radical) under a name that makes it difficult to argue against.

EBM is most popularly defined as the "conscientious and judicious use of current best evidence in the healthcare of individuals and populations" (Sackett et al., 1996b). EBM's influential doctrine first appeared in the *Journal of the American Medical Association* as a brief polemic authored by the Evidence Based Medicine Working Group:

> *A new paradigm for medical practice is emerging. Evidence based medicine de-emphasizes intuition, unsystematic clinical experience, and pathophysiologic rationale as sufficient grounds for clinical decision-making and stresses the examination of evidence from clinical research. EBM requires new skills of the physician, including efficient literature searching and the application of the formal rules of evidence (Evidence Based Medicine Working Group [EBMWG], 1992).*

EBM rose quickly into prominence in medicine, with virtually every area of healthcare now subscribing to the evidence based mantra. This is a considerable feat for a discipline that is described in the EBM manifesto as largely reliant on conventions and habits of thought and practice.

Yet amidst the hubris, there is a sort of obviousness to EBM that has prompted critics to charge EBM with offering "nothing new" (Benitez-Bribiesca, 1999):

> *"Evidence based medicine," one chemist said to me, "What other kind of medicine could there possibly be?" and a consultant physician said gruffly: "We have always practiced evidence based medicine" (Hope, 1995).*[1]

The EBM pioneers equivocated on the movement's innovation and conservatism. It was described as both a "new paradigm" (EBMWG, 1992) and a historically-supported approach "whose philosophical origins extend back to mid-19th century Paris and earlier" (Sackett et al., 1996b). Yet it will be demonstrated in this chapter that although EBM is not best understood as a new "paradigm" or a radical departure from biomedicine, it offers methodological innovation that has shifted how we pursue, collect, and evaluate medical knowledge.

Beginning with a historical account of the origins of EBM, a focus on three key methodological innovations employed by EBM will be used to advance the argument that EBM's original contribution to medicine, or what separates EBM from other approaches, is the priority it gives to certain forms of evidence, specifically evidence from randomized controlled trials. EBM offers a shift in the sort of evidence that is most highly valued for diagnosis, therapy, and prognosis questions, as heavy emphasis is placed on experimental controls and quantified measures, thus diminishing the previous status of clinical experience and observational studies significantly. This commitment represents not only methodological change, but also a novel regard of the reliability of various forms of medical knowledge. EBM offers a new answer to medicine's fundamental normative question: how ought we to practice medicine?

2. The origins of evidence-based medicine

The origins of the evidence-based medicine movement are traceable back to a series of lectures given by epidemiologist Archie Cochrane in the early 1970s, where he argued that many popularly used medical practices were of unknown or questionable safety and efficacy (Ashcroft, 2004). In these lectures, which were later compiled in *Effectiveness and Efficiency: Random Reflections on Health Services* (Cochrane, 1972), he detailed the injury, waste, and failure to improve care that ensued from widespread acceptance and use of unestablished medical interventions. He maintained that treatments should be evaluated using unbiased methods like the randomized controlled trial, and that health care professionals should regularly update their knowledge base (Ashcroft, 2004). Aschcroft has noted the strong ethical imperative behind Cochrane's recommendations, as they were rooted in concern to do no harm, to do one's best for one's patients, and to do so justly by eliminating waste (Ashcroft, 2004).

Cochrane's programmatic outline was revitalized in 1990 by a group of professors of clinical epidemiology, medical informatics, and biostatistics at McMaster University in Canada, who called themselves the "Evidence Based Medicine Working Group". They introduced the phrase "Evidence Based Medicine" in a ubiquitous 1992 manifesto as a "new paradigm" in medical education and practice (EBMWG, 1992). In the document, the ethical promise was made that the virtuous clinician "whose practice is based on an understanding of the

---

[1] Hope is a supporter of EBM who maintains that one sign of a movement being important is when its detractors indignantly maintain that it is nothing new.

underlying evidence will provide superior patient care" (EBMWG, 1992). While the ethical imperative to improve patient care remained central, the promise to decrease medical uncertainty by systematic evaluation of the efficacy of current practices was particularly appealing to health care administrators and policy analysts facing a crisis situation with respect to escalating healthcare costs and spending. Added to the gamut of methodologies for data collection and analysis first recommended by Cochrane was the use of emerging information technologies to synthesize the large quantities of published studies, proliferate information, and increase accessibility. The combined picture of EBM as ethically driven to improve patient care, fiscally responsible, and technologically up-to-date likely drove the rapid integration of the movement into medicine, where just over twenty years since the Evidence Based Medicine Working Group formed, EBM is now common parlance within health care. Academic centres and journals dedicated to EBM's advancement have been established with much fanfare, and the evidence-based movement has stretched beyond the health sciences to business management (Kovner et al., 2000; Kovner & Rundall, 2006), public health (McGuire, 2005), speech pathology (Reilly et al., 2004), occupational therapy (Von Zweck, 1999) social work (Cournoyer, 2004; Howard et al., 2003; Grinnell & Unrau, 2010), education (Council for Exceptional Children, 2011; Horner et al., 2005; Slavin, 2002), and other social science disciplines. It is even generating attention as a promising new approach to bioethics ("evidence-based ethics") (Roberts, 2000; Strech, 2008; the rare criticism is found in Goldenberg, 2005). The term "evidence-based everything" has been used to describe the enthusiasm for this movement (Mykhalovskiy & Weir, 2004).

3. What's new about EBM?

Despite the fanfare, it is not immediately obvious that EBM offers something new to medical practice. In response to EBM's demand that medical decisions ought to be based on stringent empirical evidence, critics ask, hasn't modern medicine *always* been evidence-based? Quite surely, by being founded on natural science, biomedicine has always been grounded in the empirical sciences, which bases its claims on observational evidence.

The critics are correct to think that EBM's empirical commitments are not new to medicine's ideal practices (regardless of whether or not they are actually practiced). However, proponents have denied the charge that EBM is "old hat" (Sackett et al., 1996b), and have even been grandiose in their descriptions of EBM as being a "new paradigm" promising to "revolutionize" medicine (EBMWG, 1992). This description suggests the evidence based approach to offer something radically different from previous approaches, and so it is worth investigating this alleged paradigm change.

3.1 Is EBM a new paradigm?

To illustrate the unique workings of EBM, the new paradigm of medicine, the Evidence Based Medicine Working Group presented the following clinical scenario:

> *A junior medical resident working in a teaching hospital admits a 43-year old previously well man who experiences a witnessed grand mal seizure. He had never had a seizure before and had not had any recent head trauma...Findings on physical examination are normal. The patient is given a loading dose of phenytoin intravenously and the drug is continued orally. A computed tomographic head scan is completely normal, and an electroencephalogram shows only non-*

specific findings. The patient is very concerned about his risk of seizure recurrence. How might the resident proceed (EBMWG, 1992)?

The Working Group explain that the resident practicing *"the way of the past"* (pre-EBM) would consult the senior resident, who, supported in his view by the attending physician, informs her that the risk of seizure recurrence is high, although its precise risk factor is unknown to him. He instructs the resident to relay this information and the related precautions to the patient. The resident does as she is told and the patient, still fearful, is discharged (EBMWG, 1992). In *"the way of the future"*, however, the EBM-trained resident asks herself whether she knows the prognosis of a first seizure and, realizing that she does not, proceeds to the library and conducts a literature search on the *Grateful Med* (now *PubMed*) search engine. Her search on the medical subject headings "epilepsy", "prognosis", and "recurrence" retrieves twenty-five titles, of which one is deemed by the resident to be directly relevant. Exercising the critical appraisal skills that she learned in medical school, she reviews the paper, deems the study and its conclusions to be valid, and returns to her patient after only thirty minutes. She conveys the risk of recurrence over time post-incident, and recommends follow-up with his family physician. The patient leaves "with a clear idea of his likely prognosis" (EBMWG, 1992).

In their comparative analysis of EBM and its biomedical predecessor, Sehon and Stanley argue that the EBM programmatic literature's likening of its approach to a Kuhnian paradigm shift is a gross exaggeration (Sehon & Stanley, 2003). The authors contend that EBM is not a new paradigm because Kuhn described such a large-scale scientific revolution as involving dramatic changes of worldview and even a different world in which scientists must operate (Kuhn, 1996). A Kuhnian paradigm is an "entire constellation of beliefs, values, techniques, and so on shared by the members of a given community" (Kuhn, 1996). The new paradigm will be *incommensurable,* to some extent, with the previous paradigm, a condition that is not met with the evidence based approach in comparison to biomedicine's "basic science approach", which involves "studying the physiological mechanisms of the body and the biochemical properties of drugs" (Sehon & Stanley, 2003).

When EBM is suggested to be a new paradigm, this fosters the impression that an entire set of beliefs, values, and techniques are being discarded, "and that the whole world of medical research and clinical practice is completely different than it was in the days before EBM" (Sehon & Stanley, 2003). This impression is certainly false. Furthermore, the language of paradigms suggests that health care practitioners must make a "stark choice" between EBM and "traditional" biomedicine, where one can "accept the new regime and completely reject the old, or defensively hold onto the old and dismiss EBM entirely" (Sehon & Stanley, 2003). Aside from not being a productive atmosphere in which to hold a critical debate about EBM, this polarization exaggerates the merits, demerits, and differences between EBM and its biomedical "predecessor".

Numerous commentators have characterized the EBM debate as dredging up the hoary "art versus science" dispute regarding the nature of modern clinical medicine. The critics worry that EBM overemphasizes the latter at the expense of the former. Sullivan and MacNaughton, for example, comment that

> *the doctor does not deal with illnesses alone but with people who are ill, and for each individual the illness is unique in terms of his or her experience of it and in its presentation to the doctor (Sullivan & MacNaughton, 1996).*

Understanding the unique circumstances of the individual case is thought to involve a form of practical knowledge or judgment quite different from the *technical* knowledge offered by EBM. The "grey zones" of practice (Naylor, 1995), that is, areas where the evidence from randomized trials about risk-benefit ratios of competing clinical options is incomplete, inconclusive, or contradictory and so clinical judgment must be relied on,[2] are repeatedly argued to be missing from EBM's formulaic knowledge base (Tanenbaum, 1993). Indeed, EBM struggles to account for the interpretive dimensions of clinical care, as evidence-based decisionmaking is largely an effort to standardize and rationalize the application of evidence to clinical care. It is no wonder that critics fail to be persuaded by EBM's conciliatory efforts, such as making the first principle of EBM "*evidence is never enough*" in the authoritative *Users' Guides to the Medical Literature* textbook (Guyatt & Rennie, 2002). It is also worth asking: if evidence is not the fundamental base of medicine, are we still practicing evidence *based* medicine?

In light of these grey zones, EBM is charged with creating and sustaining the idea that *evidence* and *practice* are opposing concepts (Pope 2003; Wood et al., 1998). Other dualisms reinforced in the EBM literature include technical vs. experiential/intuitive knowledge, empirical vs. theoretical knowledge, evidence based vs. patient-centred care, and, of course, EBM vs. its biomedical predecessor, which is inappropriately referred to as "traditional medicine".[3] Adherence to these artificial bifurcations seems to misdirect the EBM debate, as they promote undue polarization between EBM and its biomedical alternatives. For instance, the references to pre-EBM as "traditional medicine" in some of the early EBM programmatic literature (EBMWG, 1992; Sackett et al, 1996b) is an obvious misnomer, as the term typically refers to folk and alternative healing practices. The selection of this inappropriate term was presumably deliberate, as it permitted the EBM originators to emphasize what they alleged to be the widespread tendency of clinical medicine to operate without sufficient evidentiary support to establish the efficacy of their practices. Pre-EBM biomedicine was therefore "traditional" insofar as it is unscientific or at least insufficiently scientific. Some support for this claim has been found in the phenomenon of small area variations of healthcare practice among different geographical regions (Parchman, 1995). However invoking "traditional medicine" is polemical (and distracting) in its misrepresentation of biomedicine, as it cannot account for biomedicine's modern scientific framework, its significant technological advances and achievements, and, of course, EBM's ties to the biomedical tradition.

Despite not invoking revolution (or comparable large-scale upheaval) in medical practice, it will now be demonstrated that EBM brings something new to medicine. The critics who deny this claim likely do so because they misunderstand EBM to be asking for no more than rigorous empirical research in medicine. But the term "evidence based" amounts to much more. While the evidence based approach certainly does call for rigorous empirical research in medicine, this call is accompanied by novel accounts of what counts as valid evidence

---

[2] Among the procedures cited by Naylor to be in the "grey zone" are: carotid endarterectomy, upper gastrointestinal (GI) endoscopy, hysterectomy, and percutaneous transluminal coronary angioplasty. Randomized controlled trials have been done in these areas, but the results have not produced unequivocal conclusions.

[3] Accompanying these imposed bifurcations are, of course, efforts at integration, such as "evidence-based patient centred care" (Borgmeyer, 2005), and "evidence-based patient choice" (Hope, 1996; Edwards & Elwyn, 2001; Parker, 2001). The literature also includes an effort to overcome (or possibly deny) the evidence/judgment divide (Downie et al., 2000).

and what qualifies as the most rigorous methods of empirical research. Rather than a revolution or paradigm change, EBM represents an important *shift* in biomedical thinking and practice that is a significant alternative to its biomedical predecessor. Specifically, EBM offers a shift in the sort of evidence that is most highly valued for diagnostics, prognostics, and therapeutics, in its emphasis on experimental controls and quantitative research, which undermines previous regard of clinical experience and observational studies significantly (Sehon & Stanley, 2003). At minimum, this shift is signified by a change from a medical model grounded in basic science to a novel statistically-based medicine (Henry, 2006). EBM's hierarchy of evidence is at the service of outcomes research, which uses a cluster of statistical and epidemiological methods for analyzing the therapeutic effectiveness of clinical interventions (Gifford, 1996). This commitment to highly controlled data and methods of statistical analysis that were previously used only for population-based research (such as public health) represents not only methodological change, but also a novel regard of the reliability of various forms of medical knowledge.

4. The novel contents of EBM

The unique content offered to medicine by EBM remains difficult for many to grasp. Hardly anyone can disagree with the goal of getting clinicians to make "conscientious, explicit, and judicious use of current best evidence" for decisions in patient care. Any expressions of doubt about EBM activities are usually greeted with vigorous accusations of disregarding "today's harsh realities", or ignoring "what happens in clinical medicine" (Sackett et al., 1996a). Furthermore, critics are frequently denounced for erroneous beliefs that EBM only uses evidence from randomized controlled trials, that it involves "merely the mindless application of the results of megatrials", and that "other forms of evidence are heavily discounted" (Rosenberg & Donald, 1995). Feinstein and Horwitz have wisely suggested that much of the confusion surrounding what EBM actually stands for lies in the distinction between the contents of EBM itself and its application in clinical practice. It is only when this distinction is blurred that many clinicians claim EBM to offer "nothing new" (Feinstein & Horwitz, 1997). Many practitioners have seen little novelty in EBM because they regularly assemble evidence, develop clinical judgment, read medical literature, attend medical meetings, and have discussions with one another. These activities seem entirely compatible with the statement that the practice of EBM consists of "integrating individual clinical expertise with the best available external clinical evidence from systematic research" (Sackett et al., 1996b). The activities surrounding the practice of EBM also seems fairly standard, as the data informing evidence-based practice "is not restricted to randomized trials and meta-analyses" (Sackett et al., 1996b). It contains "clinically relevant research, often from the basic sciences of medicine" and it includes studies of diagnostic tests, prognostic markers, and "the efficacy and safety of the therapeutic, rehabilitative and preventive regimes" (Sackett et al., 1996b). With this description of what is done when EBM is *practiced* and with the overt acknowledgement by the EBM originators that EBM is rooted in the medical thought of mid-nineteenth century France, specifically "the call for external evidence expressed in Paris 150 years ago by Louis, Bichat and Magendie" (Sackett et al., 1997), clinicians can easily conclude that EBM is not particularly novel, and may wonder why it has stirred so much fuss and controversy (Feinstein & Horwitz, 1997).

The novelty lies, however, in the organization and privileging of information. While a wide range of evidentiary sources are permitted in evidence-based practice, the evidence collected for EBM itself is confined almost exclusively to RCTs and meta-analyses of those trials. The RCT is consistently ranked at the top of the hierarchy of evidence, thus confirming the former's privileged position (Feinstein & Horwitz, 1997). For instance, Sackett et al. maintain that for questions of therapy,

> *we should try to avoid the nonexperimental approaches, since they routinely lead to false-positive conclusions about efficacy...The randomized trial, and especially the systematic review of several randomized trials...has become the "gold standard" (Sackett et al, 1996b, as cited in Feinstein & Horwitz, 1997).*

The analysis in the next three sections will further examine the novel contents of EBM captured in its methodological privileging of (1) the hierarchy of evidence, (2) the randomized controlled trial, and (3) outcomes measures.

4.1 The hierarchy of evidence

The hierarchy of evidence captures EBM's basic methodological and epistemic commitments in a fairly straightforward ranking of methods. EBM proponents strongly hold that the trustworthiness or validity of evidence is a function of the design of the study from which the evidence is obtained (Sackett, 1989, 1997; Sackett et al., 1991; Solomon & McLeod, with the Canadian Task Force on the Periodic Health Examination, 1994), and so the desire to use only the "best evidence from clinical research" in the management of individual patients (Sackett et al, 1996b, 1997) has resulted in intricate classificatory schemes for ranking the value of different types of studies. Among the numerous published formulations, there is a consistent placement of randomized controlled trials or the systematic review of these trials at the top, retrospective studies well down the list, and clinical anecdotes are seen as providing little if any evidence for the value of intervention (see Fig. 1).

A Hierarchy of Strength of Evidence for Treatment Decisions

- N of 1 randomized controlled trial
- Systematic reviews of randomized controlled trials
- Single randomized trial
- Systematic review of observational studies addressing patient-important outcomes
- Single observational study addressing patient-important outcomes
- Physiologic studies (studies addressing blood pressure, cardiac output, exercise capacity, bone density, and so forth)
- Unsystematic clinical observations

Fig. 1. *Users' Guide to Medical Literature* hierarchy of evidence (Rennie & Guyatt, 2002)

While EBM has evolved over time, most notably in its self-regard from a (polemical) "new paradigm" to a more tempered technique for clinicians to manage vast quantities of research information (for example, Haynes, 2002), the core belief that evidence belongs in fixed hierarchical order with the systematic review of randomized controlled trials always on top remains unshaken (Upshur et al., 2001). In the evaluation of treatment effects, for example, a large, well-designed, randomized trial is considered more reliable than those findings from non-randomized prospective or retrospective studies (Sackett, 1997). Similar schemes have been developed for the ranking of evidence in other clinical categories such as prognosis, aetiology, and diagnosis (Centre for Evidence-Based

Medicine, 2006; Sackett et al., 1997). At the bottom of each of these clinical scales is evidence obtained from case reports and personal experience.

The logic behind the ranking of evidence is simple: randomization is the best method for distinguishing between the effects of active treatment from the effects of known and unknown potentially biasing influences (Peto & Baigent, 1988). It follows that we should make every effort to identify and catalogue these studies. And this is exactly what is happening. EBM proponents initially endorsed the teaching of critical analysis skills in medical schools so that physicians could properly assess the quality of a study (EBMWG, 1992). The hierarchy of evidence is one of the tools used in this task. It was quickly realized, however, that more advanced informatics were needed in order for clinicians to manage the massive amount of research data available. The Cochrane Collaboration has undertaken the monumental task of identifying and evaluating well over a million randomized controlled trials (U.S. Cochrane Center, 2002). Systematic reviews and meta-analyses of randomized trials in specific areas of medicine are now widely available on EBM databases and in EBM journals.

The privileging of "hard" evidence—the quantified data generated by randomized controlled trials—over knowledge generated from clinical experience (EBMWG, 1992) and qualitative measures (Gray, 1997) speaks to an epistemic distrust of subjective or personal experience, which cannot guard against biasing influences. Methodologies like blinding, randomization, placebo-control, the use of large subject populations, and replication of results serve to abstract from values to reveal empirical facts. Of the types of trials available, clinical trials offer the strongest and clearest support for any claim that a treatment is effective because they allow scientists to control extraneous variables and test one factor at a time (Schick & Vaughn, 2002). The hierarchy of evidence is, by the founders' own admission, based on levels of certainty, where the quantified and the scientific forms of evidence are placed on top because they are understood to be most resistant to sceptical refutation (Sackett et al., 1991).

The central goal behind the EBM movement is quality of care, and this goal serves as the grounds for encouraging medical practice that utilizes the latest and best evidence. Evidence-based practices, including the ranking of evidence, are thought to enhance effective and efficient clinical decision-making. But, critics argue, "effectiveness" need not be limited to clinical- or cost-effectiveness. It could also refer to patient-based outcomes indicating satisfaction with the treatment provided. The hierarchy prioritizes evidence of clinical effectiveness and necessarily excludes subjective perceptions (Malterud, 1995, 2001; Rogers 2002). Yet patient narratives and the interpretive features of clinical practice are thought by many to be crucial features of quality healthcare (Greenhalgh & Hurwitz, 1998; Greenhalgh, 1999; Malterud 2001; Silva et al., 2011).

4.2 Randomized controlled trials: The "gold standard" of medical research

The methodological debates that make up the bulk of the EBM literature revolve around the general question whether or not the refined focus on clinical evidence (as prioritized in the EBM hierarchy of knowledge), or the search for secure knowledge in general, improves our ability to decipher best practices and therefore prescribe the most effective treatments. Alternatively, the methods may leave out too many important features of clinical care that are not readily measurable through evidence-based approaches. This leads to the important further question of whether the randomized controlled trial rightfully deserves the title of "gold standard".

Regarded as a maverick among his peers, Cochrane strongly promoted the controversial view that randomized controlled trials offer the best test for the effects of medical interventions and could thereby correct ineffectiveness and even harms perpetrated by contemporary medical practice (this was another heretical claim) (Pope, 2003). With time, this view came to be accepted and randomized trials became "a yardstick by which other sources of information were judged and ranked within a hierarchy of evidence" (Pope, 2003). The introduction of randomized trials to medical research has been credited by Iain Chalmers, one of the original founders of the Cochrane Collaboration who was knighted in 2000 for his activism in cumulating evidence in medical research, and others for revolutionizing therapeutic development and increasing the life expectancy of patients from three to seven years over the past half century (Chalmers, 1998). When substantial uncertainty exists about treatment effects, it is widely thought to be not only scientifically correct to answer it in a study with the smallest amount of built-in bias, but also most ethical to expose patients to alternative treatment options based on chance only and not upon the biased opinion of a physician (Edwards et al., 1998; Frazier & Mosteller, 1995; Freedman, 1997; Lilford & Jackson, 1995).

Many EBM critics point to the "experiential nature" of medical practice for being not only inextricable from but also inappropriately maligned by the evidence based approach (Tanenbaum 1993; Williams & Garner, 2002). However, supporters of EBM insist that experiential knowledge is worth minimizing because experience allows for the repetition of mistakes. EBM proponents point to the data available suggesting human fallibility and bias in drawing conclusions based on uncontrolled experience (Dawson & Arkes, 1987; MacCoun, 1998). Others argue that investigators with relationships or experience with a subject form expectations with respect to treatment outcomes that make them less able to produce objective reviews of scientific evidence than non-experts trained in critical appraisal of evidence (Oxman & Guyatt, 1993). A logical deductive framework for interpretation of evidence is therefore argued to be needed if we are to avoid practicing medicine based on uncontrolled experience, which may do more harm than good (Sackett, 1989). The nature of research is meant to reduce uncertainty, even if it cannot be completely eliminated. Yet what randomized controlled trials gain in experimental certainty (internal validity), they lose in applicability to the clinical context (external validity) (Cartwright, 2007). The EBM hierarchy indicates a strong presumption in favour of internal validity in experimental design.

The randomized controlled trial design is better geared for certain kinds of intervention questions than others. These trials are ideal for the direct comparison between simple treatments such as two single drugs, and so the pronounced "hegemony of the double-blind randomized controlled trial" (Charlton, 1991) can both undermine research into the use of complex interventions and result in a failure to meet the complex needs of individual patients. Regarding the former, the critics worry that because randomized controlled trial design is increasingly favoured, and because the expectation to provide "best evidence" of effectiveness before implementing interventions is growing, complex interventions are by default less likely to be supported over time (DeVries & Lemmens, 2006). As a result, behavioural, psychosocial, community based, and multiple-component interventions lose out in favour of individual patient-based treatments (Dieppe, 1998; Tallon et al., 2000) and resultant public health policy-setting increasingly focuses on individuals rather than on groups (Davey-Smith et al., 2001). Speaking more abstractly, numerous philosophers of science deny that there is any universal method in science, randomized trial or otherwise (Cartwright, 2007; Urbach, 1993; Worrall, 2002).

In the arena of individual patient care, critics argue that because EBM guidelines are derived from controlled trials of simplified clinical situations using criteria that often exclude other complicating serious conditions, the evidence may not be applicable to complex clinical situations. The "gold standard" of clinical research is widely thought to have a problem of generalizability of its results to individual patient care (Britton et al., 1998; Culpepper & Gilbert, 1999; Feinstein & Horwitz, 1997). Even Cochrane recognized that while the RCT can measure effectiveness, its results may not be directly replicable in clinical practice (Cochrane, 1972), and so Dingwall et al. seem correct in their suggestion that Cochrane's ideas have been used somewhat selectively in EBM (Dingwall et al., 1988, as cited in Pope, 2003). The problem of generalizability begins with the narrow eligibility criteria for randomized trials, which limit conclusions about a treatment's effectiveness to patients who fulfill those criteria (Feinstein & Horwitz, 1997). To demonstrate optimal efficacy, randomized controlled trials often use relatively homogenous subject populations (Djulbegovic et al., 2000). Patients excluded from such trials can differ substantially from study patients in a variety of ways that could influence treatment outcomes (i.e. disease severity, comorbid conditions, gender, race) (Britton et al., 1998; Tanenbaum, 1995). Furthermore, the time periods covered in clinical trials and the measures used to assess outcomes frequently differ from those used to assess the success of a therapy in actual practice. In an effort to be efficient, clinical trials typically use the shortest time possible for determining valid results, employing surrogate endpoints rather than clinically relevant outcomes. Surrogate endpoints are physiological or biochemical markers that can be ascertained quickly and taken to be predictive of clinically meaningful endpoints—such as how a patient feels, functions, or survives—that take much longer to observe. They are "surrogate" insofar as they are outcome measures that are not of direct practical importance but are believed to reflect outcomes that are clinically relevant. For example, cholesterol studies frequently use cholesterol reduction as a surrogate for reduced mortality. Direct demonstration of mortality reduction requires lengthy trials using large subject populations, while cholesterol reduction is known to be strongly associated with mortality benefits, and can be measured easily in smaller numbers of patients. Similarly, blood pressure is not directly important to patients but it is often used as an outcome in clinical trials because it is a risk factor for stroke and heart attacks (Bandolier, n.d.).

Yet the requirement that surrogate endpoints reliably predict the overall effect of the clinical outcome frequently fails in practice (Fleming & DeMets, 1996). The disease process can affect the clinical outcome through several causal pathways that are not mediated by the surrogate. Therefore the effect of the intervention on these pathways will be different from the effect on the surrogate (Fleming & DeMets, 1996). It is more likely, however, that "the intervention affects the clinical outcome by unintended, unanticipated, and unrecognized mechanisms of action that operate independently of the disease process" (Fleming & DeMets, 1996). Fleming and DeMets argue that surrogate endpoints frequently mislead regarding the actual effects that treatments have on health outcomes. For instance, although lipid levels are widely seen to be important predictors of cardiovascular-related mortality, there is debate over the relationship between lipid lowering and reduction in overall mortality. The Coronary Drug Project in the 1970's showed clofibrate and niacin to decrease cholesterol levels, however neither agent reduced total mortality (Fleming & DeMets, 1996).

Taken together, the numerous controls utilized to guard against bias and promote efficiency in medical research limits the relevancy of, and may even distort, the "best evidence from clinical research" in the management of individual patients. While there are differences of opinion regarding the challenges posed in making clinical evidence applicable, EBM fails to engage significantly with this problem. EBM's penchant for methodological rigour may be at odds with the ad hoc nature of clinical practice. Tanenbaum has suggested that the precision of "best evidence" is fundamentally irreconcilable with its clinical relevance, given the particularity of patients and the significant improvisational dimensions of clinical practice (Tanenbaum, 1995). Shaughnessy et al. refer to this improvisational feature as "clinical jazz" (Shaughnessy et al., 1998). The debate over randomized controlled trials highlight that the problem of evidence in EBM does not only concern what knowledge is missing from the evidence based decisionmaking framework, but also the nature of the knowledge that *does* enter into consideration.

4.3 Outcomes measures: Clinical effectiveness and the quality movement in medicine

EBM was introduced to healthcare in the wake of what has been famously described as the "third revolution" in health care (Relman, 1988),[4] a turn toward assessment and accountability in light of escalating health care costs creating a "crisis" situation in health care spending throughout the industrialized world. Patients and payers widely subscribed to a "waste theory" that described physicians wasting healthcare money on poorly performing diagnostics and treatments (Tanenbaum, 1994a). Furthermore, the documentation of notable geographical variations in practice that could not be explained by local organizational and financial arrangements caused alarm (Clancy & Eisenberg, 1988). Health care advocates wanted the consistent practice of only the best health care interventions. The "best" was determined by the "end results" or "outcomes" of medical practice. The urgency with which the public demanded that physicians pay attention to medical outcomes led to what soon became known as the "outcomes movement" in health policy (Epstein, 1990). Evaluating clinical effectiveness was seen as a fiscally responsible means of only financing the most promising therapies and research. EBM facilitated the clinical data that outcomes research requires in order to evaluate best practices.

Outcomes research refers to all activity directed towards the assessment of outcomes, analysis of effectiveness, and quality assurance (Epstein, 1990). It uses statistical analysis of clinical data to determine associations between particular therapeutic interventions and particular results (Tanenbaum, 1994a). Unlike laboratory research which measures definable clinical events like lipid lowering or blood pressure, outcomes research can employ patient-derived endpoints, the outcomes that patients care about (Clancy & Eisenberg, 1988). Common themes in outcomes research are: safety, effectiveness, equity, efficiency, timeliness, and patient centeredness (Institute of Medicine, 2001). The benefits of outcomes research to healthcare include better informed patients and providers, the development of clinical guidelines that reflect those assessments, and wiser purchasing of health care technologies (Agency for Health Care Research and Quality, n.d.). This move towards

[4] Relman later lamented that this "third revolution" was never realized due to lack of government initiative by any of the US governmental administrations elected since the 1988 writing of his editorial (Relman, 2009).

accountability is supposed to serve as a rational basis for decision making and, by extension, make medical care more efficient.

The outcomes movement argues for the primacy of probabilistic knowledge derived from statistical studies for medical practice and the vigorous adoption of this position within health care indicates a radical shift in medical rationality (Tanenbaum, 1994a). Polychronis et al., for example, regard the ascendancy of EBM as the triumph of statistics over clinical common sense based on deterministic reasoning (Polychronis et al., 1996). Clinical epidemiology, the application of epidemiologic and biometric methods to direct patient care (Sackett, 1969), is now held by some to be a basic medical science (Sackett et al., 1991). EBM distinguishes itself from pre-evidence based biomedicine by its orientation toward outcomes research, while biomedicine is more dependent on bench science. Biomedical research employs laboratory science that aims to understand the causal relationship between an intervention and a desired effect, whereby therapeutic efficacy can then be inferred. EBM seeks to generate probabilistic knowledge regarding what is likely to work for whatever reason (Tanenbaum, 1994a). John Wennberg, director of the Centre for Evaluative Clinical Science at Dartmouth Medical School, regards biomedical science to be at the service of evaluative science in treatment decisionmaking. He argues that biomedicine generates new technologies, while evaluative science provides the crucial data linking treatments to outcomes (Wennberg, 1992).

The consistent placement of the randomized controlled trial at the top of the EBM hierarchy of evidence is better understood in light of the biomedical versus evidence-based distinction, as this research method serves the objectives of outcomes research by appearing to bracket out a whole range of scientifically and epistemologically difficult questions about why treatments do or not work (Ashcroft, 2002). For instance, rather than determining the properties that enable or hinder an intervention's success, randomized controlled trials establish efficacy by comparing the outcomes of the experimental arm with those found in a similar subject population receiving a comparator intervention. Eliminating bench science's focus on determining *why* a treatment works or not through appeal to deeper biological theory has certain advantages for healthcare decision-making (Ashcroft 2002; Gifford 1996).[5] Definitive biological explanation has not always led to safe or beneficial treatment of actual patients. The randomized trial "acts as a practical filter permitting the calibration of scientific good ideas against clinical reality (however that is constructed)" (Ashcroft, 2002). By comparing two or more competing courses of treatment (including placebo), the RCT "offers a technique for dispute resolution within medicine: where there is discord, let a trial be" (Ashcroft, 2002).

Because EBM and outcomes research are closely allied, the concerns regarding the latter are similar to those launched against the former. The task of outcomes research, to solve the problems of quality and cost that beset the healthcare system and to do so by scientific rather than political means, raises the concern about the tenability of value-free measures (Goldenberg 2006). Furthermore, Tanenbaum's account of the "epistemological politics" of the US outcomes movement (Tanenbaum, 1994a) brings into question whether this research can ever be so benign that it merely informs decision makers and helps them make better decisions (Sage, 1994). The championing of probabilistic knowledge to improve clinical practice is argued to replace subjective professional judgment with micromanagement by insurance companies and government (Tanenbaum 1993, 1995).

[5] Of course there are several ways in which "does it work?" can be construed (Ashcroft et al., 1997).

While Tanenbaum is accused of pandering to the fears of physicians and other professionals who perceive outcomes research to be a threat to autonomous practice (Cangialose, 1994), her criticisms are not against outcomes research *per se*, as she recognizes the usefulness of statistical analysis in evaluating medical care. Her target is rather the outcomes *movement*, the "organized effort of one research community and its champions to gain special privilege for statistical evidence, to consider it the only true evidence of medical effectiveness, and to predicate an accountable health care system on physicians' adherence to norms of practice derived from outcomes studies" (Tanenbaum, 1994b). Similar to EBM, the critics find utility in outcomes research for improving patient care, but they question its near-hegemonic status in influential health policy and administrative circles.

5. Conclusion

While this analysis dampens some of the hubris surrounding the evidence-based movement, it highlights the significant methodological innovation that EBM has brought to medicine. The evidence based approach is marked by the flourishing relationship that the evaluative sciences and informatics, once solely the domain of business and managerial studies, now have with medicine. Eliciting EBM's place within the "quality movement" (Bodenheimer, 1999) captures a shift in medical rationality and knowledge away from previous incarnations of biomedicine by way of EBM's insistent epistemological privileging of standardized information over judgment, quantified measurement over experience, and epidemiology over bench science.

6. References

Agency for Health Care Research and Quality (n.d). Outcomes Research Fact Sheet. In: *U.S. Department for Health & Human Services*, October 2011, Available from: http://www.ahrq.gov/clinic/outfact.htm

Ashcroft, R. E. (2002). What is clinical effectiveness? *Studies in the History and Philosophy of Science Part C: Biological and Biomedical Sciences*, Vol. 33, No. 2, (July 2002), pp. 219-233, 0039-3681

Ashcroft, R. E. (2004). Current epistemological problems in evidence-based medicine. *Journal of Medical Ethics* 30, 2, (April 2004), pp. 131-135, 0306-6800

Ashcroft, R. E., Chawick, D. W., Clark, S. R., Edwards, R. H., Frith, L. & Hutton, J. L. (1997). Implications of socio-cultural contexts for the ethics of clinical trials." *Health Technology Assessment*, Vol. 1, No. 9, (July 1997), pp. 1-65, 1366-5278

Bandolier. (n.d.). Surrogate Endpoints. In: *Bandolier Glossary of Terms*, October 2011, Available from: http://www.medicine.ox.ac.uk/bandolier/booth/glossary/surrog.html

Benitez-Bribiesca, L. (1999). Evidence-based medicine: A new paradigm? *Archives of Medical Research*, 30, 2, (March-April 1999), pp. 77-79, 0188-4409

Bodenheimer, T. (1999). The movement for improved quality of health care. *New England Journal of Medicine* 340, 6, (February 1999), pp. 488-492, 0028-4793

Borgmeyer, C. (2005). Guideline showcases AAFP's commitment to evidence-based, patient-centered care. *Annals of Family Medicine*, Vol. 3, No. 4, (July-August 2005), pp. 378-380, 1544-1709

Britton, A., McKee, M., Black, N., McPherson, K., Sanderson, C. & Bain, C. (1998). Choosing between randomized and non-randomized studies: A systematic review. *Health Technology Assessment*, Vol. 2, No. 13, (May 1998), pp. 1-124, 1366-5278

Cangialose, C. B. (1994). Outcomes research [letter]. *New England Journal of Medicine*, Vol. 330, No. 6, (February 1994), p. 435, 0028-4793

Carr-Hill, R. (1995). Welcome? To the brave new world of evidence-based medicine. *Social Science & Medicine*, 41, 11, (December 1995), pp. 1467-1468, 02779536

Cartwright, N. (2007). Are RCTs the gold standard? *Biosocieties*, Vol. 2, No. 1, (March 2007), pp. 11-20, 1745-8552

Centre for Evidence-Based Medicine. (2006). Levels of evidence and grades of recommendation. In: *Centre for Evidence-Based Medicine*, October 2011, Available from: http://www.cebm.net/levels_of_evidence.asp

Chalmers, I. (1998). Unbiased, relevant, and reliable assessments in health care. *British Medical Journal*, Vol. 317, No. 7167, (October 1998), pp. 1167-1168, 0959-8138

Charlton, B. (1991). Medical practice and the double-blind, randomized controlled trial. *British Journal of General Practice* ,Vol. 41, No. 350, pp. 335-336, 0960-1643

Clancy, C. M. & Eisenberg, J. M. (1988). Outcomes research: Measuring the end results of health care. *Science*, Vol. 282, No. 5387, (October 1988), pp. 245-246, 0036-8075

Cochrane, A. L. (1972). *Effectiveness and Efficiency. Random Reflections on Health Services*, Nuffield Provincial Hospitals Trust, 0900574178, London

Council for Exceptional Children. (2011). Evidence-based practice—Wanted, needed, and hard to get. In: *Council for Exceptional Children*, October 2011, Available from: http://www.cec.sped.org/AM/Template.cfm?Section=Home&CONTENTID=6515&TEMPLATE=/CM/Co ntentDisplay.cfm&CAT=none

Cournoyer, B. R. (2004). *The Evidence-Based Social Work Skills Book*, Pearson, 0205358624, Boston

Culpepper, L. & Gilbert, T. T. (1999). Evidence and ethics. *Lancet*, Vol. 353, No. 9155, (March 1999), pp. 829-831, 0140- 6736

Davey-Smith, G., Ebrahim, S., & Frankel, S. (2001). How policy informs the evidence. *British Medical Journal*, Vol. 322, No. 7286, (January 2001), pp. 184-185, 0959-8138

Dawson, N. V. & Arkes, H. R. (1987). Systematic errors in medical decision making: Judgment limitations. *Journal of General Internal Medicine*, Vol. 2, No. 3, (May-June 1987), pp. 183-187, 1525-1497

De Vries, T. & Lemmens, T. (2006). The social and cultural shaping of medical evidence: Case studies from pharmaceutical research and obstetric science. *Social Science and Medicine*, Vol. 62, No. 11, (June 2006), pp. 2694-2706, 02779536

Dieppe, P. (1998). Evidence-based medicine or medicine-based evidence? *Annals of Rheumatological Disease*, Vol. 57, No. 7, (July 1998), pp. 385-386, 0003-4967

Djulbegovic, B., Morris, L., Lyman, G. H. (2000). Evidentiary challenges to evidence-based medicine. *Journal of Evaluation in Clinical Practice*, Vol. 6, No. 2, (May 2000), pp. 99-109, 1365-2753

Downie, R. S., MacNaughton, J., & Randall, F. (2000). *Clinical Judgment: Evidence in Practice*. Oxford University Press, 0192632167, London

Edwards, A. & Elwyn, G., eds. (2001). *Evidence-Based Patient Choice: Inevitable or Impossible?* Oxford University Press, 0-19-263194-2, Oxford

Edwards, S. J. L., Lilford, R. J., Braunholtz, D. A., Jackson, J. C., Hewison, J. & Thornton, J. (1988). Ethical issues in the design and conduct of randomized controlled trials. *Health Technology Assessment*, Vol. 2, No. 15, (December 1988), pp. 1-132, 1366-5278

Epstein, A. M. (1990). The outcomes movement—will it get us where we want to go? *New England Journal of Medicine*, Vol. 323, No. 4, (July 1990), pp. 266-270, 0028-4793

Evidence-Based Medicine Working Group (EBMWG). (1992). Evidence-based medicine: A new approach to teaching the practice of medicine. *Journal of the American Medical Association*, Vol. 268, No. 17, (November 1992), pp. 2420-2425, 0098-7484

Feinstein, A. R. & Horwitz, R. I. (1997). Problems in the 'evidence' of 'evidence-based medicine'. *American Journal of Medicine*, Vol. 103, No. 6, (December 1995), pp. 529-535, 0002-9343

Fleming, T.R. & DeMets, D.L. (1996). Surrogate end points in clinical trials: Are we being misled? *Annals of Internal Medicine*, Vol. 125, No. 7, (October 1996), pp. 605-613, 0003-4819

Frazier, H. S. & Mosteller, F. (1995). *Medicine Worth Paying For: Assessing Medical Innovations*, Harvard University Press, 0-674-56362-X, Cambridge

Freedman, B. (1987). Equipoise and the ethics of clinical research. *New England Journal of Medicine*, Vol. 317, No. 3, (July 1987), pp. 141-145, 0028-4793

Gifford, F. (1996). Outcomes research: Upstream issues for downstream users. *Hastings Center Report*, Vol. 26, No. 2, (March-April 1996), pp. 38-44, 0093-0334

Goldenberg, M. J. (2005). Evidence based ethics? On evidence-based practice and the empirical turn from normative bioethics. *BMC Medical Ethics*, Vol. 6:11, (November 2005), 1472-6939

Goldenberg, M. J. (2006). On evidence and evidence-based medicine: Lessons from the philosophy of science. *Social Science and Medicine*, Vol. 62, No. 11 (June 2006), pp. 2621-2632, 0277-9536

Gray, J. A. M. (1997). *Evidence-Based Healthcare: How to Make Health Policy and Management Decisions*. Churchill Livingstone, 978-0443057212, London

Greenhalgh, T. (1999). Narrative based medicine: Narrative based medicine in an evidence based world. *British Medical Journal*, Vol. 318, No. 7179, (January 1999), pp. 323-325, 0959-8138

Greenhalgh, T. & Hurwitz, B., eds. (1998). *Narrative Based Medicine: Dialogue and Discourse in Clinical Practice*, BMJ Publishing Group, 978-0727912237, London

Grinnell, R. M. & Unrau, Y., A. (2010). *Social Work Research and Evaluation: Foundations of Evidence-Based Practice* (9th), Oxford, 978-0-19-973476-4, New York

Guyatt, G. & Rennie, D. (2002). *Users' Guides to the Medical Literature: A Manual for Evidence-Based Practice* (2nd), American Medical Association, 1-57947-174-9, Chicago

Haynes, R. B. (2002). What kind of evidence is it that evidence-based medicine advocates want health care providers and consumers to pay attention to? *BMC Health Services Research*, Vol. 2:3, (March 2006), 1472-6963

Henry, S. G. (2006). Recognizing tacit knowledge in medical epistemology. *Theoretical Medicine and Bioethics*, Vol. 27, No. 3, (May 2006), pp. 187-213, 1386-7415

Hope, T. (1995). Evidence based medicine and ethics. *Journal of Medical Ethics*, Vol. 21, No. 5, (October 1995), pp. 259-260, 0306-6800

Hope, T. (1996). *Evidence Based Patient Choice*, King's Fund Publishing, 9781857171297, London

Horner, R. H., Carr, E. G., Halle, J., McGee, G., Odom, S., & Wolery, M. (2005). The use of single-subject research to identify evidence-based practice in special education. *Exceptional Children*, Vol. 71, No. 2, pp. 165-179, 0014-4029

Howard, M. O., McMillen, C. J. & Pollio, D. E. (2003). Teaching evidence-based practice: Toward a new paradigm for social work education. *Research on Social Work Practice*, Vol. 13, No. 2, (March 2003), pp. 234-259, 1552-7581

Institute of Medicine. (2001). *Crossing the Quality Chasm: A New Health System for the 21st Century*. National Academy Press, 0-309-07280-8, Washington

Kovner, A. R., Elton, J., & Billings, J. (2000). Evidence-based management. *Frontiers of Health Services Management*, Vol. 16, No. 4, (Summer 2000), pp. 3-26, 0748-8157

Kovner, A. R. & Rundall, T. G. (2006). Evidence-based management reconsidered. *Frontiers of Health Services Management*, Vol. 22, No. 3, (Spring 2006), pp. 3-21, 0748-8157

Kuhn, T. (1996). *The Structure of Scientific Revolutions* (3rd), University of Chicago Press, 0226458083, Chicago

Lilford, R. J. & Jackson, J. (1995). Equipoise and the ethics of randomization. *Journal of the Royal Society of Medicine*, Vol. 88, No. 10, (October 1995), pp. 552-559, 0141-0768

MacCoun, R. J. 1998. Biases in the interpretation and use of research results. *Annual Review of Psychology*, Vol. 49, (February 1998), pp. 259-287, 0066-4308

Malterud, K. (1995). The legitimacy of clinical knowledge: Toward a medical epistemology embracing the art of medicine. *Theoretical Medicine*, Vol. 16, No 2, (June 1995), pp. 183-198, 1573-1200

Malterud, K. (2001). The art and science of clinical knowledge: Evidence beyond measures and numbers." *Lancet*, Vol. 358, No. 9279, (April 2001), pp. 397-400, 0140-6736

McGuire, W. L. (2005). Beyond EBM: New directions for evidence-based public health. *Perspectives in Biology and Medicine*, Vol. 48, No. 4, (Autumn 2005), pp. 557-569, 1529-8795

Mykhalovskiy, E. & Weir, L. (2004). The problem of evidence-based medicine: Directions for social medicine. *Social Science & Medicine*, Vol. 59, No. 5, (September 2004), pp. 1059-1069, 02779536

Naylor, C. D. (1995). Grey zones of clinical practice: Some limits to evidence-based medicine. *Lancet*, Vol. 345, No. 8953, (April 1995), pp. 840-842, 0140-6736

Oxman, A. D. & Guyatt, G. H. (1993). The science of reviewing research. *Annals of the New York Academy of Science*, Vol. 703, (December 1993), pp. 125-133, 0077-8923

Parchman, M. L. (1995). Small area variation analysis: A tool for primary care research. *Family Medicine*, Vol. 272, No. 4, (April 1995), pp. 272-276, 0742-3225

Parker, M. (2001). The ethics of evidence-based patient choice. *Health Expectations*, Vol. 4, No. 2, (June 2001), pp. 87-91, 1369-7625

Peto, R. & Baigent, C. (1988). Trials: The next 50 years. *British Medical Journal*, Vol. 317, No. 7167 (October 1988), pp. 1170-1171, 0959-8138

Polychronis, A., Miles, A., & Dentley, D. (1996). Evidence-based medicine: Reference? Dogma? Neologism? New orthodoxy? *Journal of Evaluation in Clinical Practice*, Vol. 2, No. 1, (February 1996), pp. 1-3, 1365-2753

Pope, C. (2003). Resisting evidence: The study of evidence-based medicine as a contemporary social movement. *Health: An Interdisciplinary Journal for the Social Study of Health, Illness, and Medicine*, Vol. 7, No. 3, (July 2003), pp. 267-282, 1363-4593

Reilly S., Douglas, J. & Oates, J. (2004). *Evidence Based Practice in Speech Pathology*, Wiley, 978-1-86156-320-0, San Francisco

Relman, A. (1988). Assessment and accountability: The third revolution in medical care. *New England Journal of Medicine*, Vol. 319, No. 18, (November 1988), pp. 1220-1222, 0028-4793

Relman, A. (2009). Assessment and accountability. *Journal of Health Services Research and Policy*, Vol. 14, No. 4, (October 2009), pp. 249-250, 1355-8196

Roberts, L. W. (2000). Evidence-based ethics and informed consent in mental illness research. *Archives of General Psychiatry*, Vol. 57, No. 6, (June 2000), pp. 540-542, 0003-990x

Rogers, W. (2002). Is there a tension between doctors' duty of care and evidence-based medicine? *Health Care Analysis*, Vol. 10, No. 3, (September 2002), pp. 277-287, 1065-3058

Rosenberg, W. M. C. & Donald, A. (1995). Evidence based medicine: An approach to clinical problem-solving. *British Medical Journal*, Vol. 310, No. 6987, (April 1995), pp. 1122-1126, 0959-8138

Sackett, D. L. (1969). Clinical epidemiology. *American Journal of Epidemiology*, Vol. 89, No. 2, (February 1969), pp. 125- 128, 1476-6256

Sackett, D. L. (1989). Rules of evidence and clinical recommendations on the use of antithrombotic agents. *Chest*, 95, 2 Suppl., (February 1989), 2S-4S, 1931-3543

Sackett, D. L. (1997). A science for the art of consensus. *Journal of the National Cancer Institute*, Vol. 89, No. 14, (July 1997), pp. 1003-1005, 1460-2105

Sackett, D. L., Haynes, R. B., Guyatt, G. H., & Tugwell, P. (1991). *Clinical Epidemiology: A Basic Science for Clinical Medicine*. Little Brown & Co., 0316765996, Boston

Sackett, D. L., Richardson, W. S., Rosenberg, W. M. C., & Haynes, R. B. (1997). *Evidence-Based Medicine: How to Practice and Teach EBM*. Churchill Livingstone, 0-443-05686-2, New York, Edinburgh, London, Madrid, Melbourne

Sackett, D. L., Rosenberg, W. M. C., Muir Gray, J. A., Haynes R. B. & Richardson W. S. (1996a). Evidence based medicine. Authors' reply. *British Medical Journal*, Vol. 313, No. 7049, (July 1996), pp. 170–171, 0959-8138

Sackett, D. L., Rosenberg, W. M. C., Muir Gray, J. A., Haynes, R. B. & Richardson, W. S. (1996b). Evidence based medicine: What it is and what it isn't. *British Medical Journal*, Vol. 312, No. 7023, (January 1996), pp. 71-72., 0959-8138

Sage, W. M. (1994). Outcomes research [letter]. *New England Journal of Medicine*, Vol. 330, No. 6, (February 1994), pp. 434-435, 0028-4793

Schick, T. & Vaughn, L. (2002). *How to Think about Weird Things: Critical Thinking for a New Age*, McGraw-Hill, 0767400135, New York

Sehon S. R. & Stanley, D. E. (2003). A philosophical analysis of the evidence-based medicine debate. *BMC Health Services Research*, Vol. 3:14, (July 2003), 1472-6963-3-14

Shaughnessy, A. F., Slawson, D. C., & Becker, L. (1998). Clinical jazz: Harmonizing clinical experience and evidence based medicine. *Journal of Family Practice*, Vol. 47, No. 6, (December 1998), pp. 425-428, 0094-3509

Silva, S. A. & Charon, R. (2011). The marriage of evidence and narrative: Scientific nurturance within clinical practice. *Journal of Evaluation in Clinical Practice*, Vol. 17, No. 4, (September 2011), pp. 585-593, 1365-2753

Slavin, R. E. (2002). Evidence-based educational policies: Transforming educational practice and research. *Educational Researcher*, Vol. 31, No. 7 (October 2002), pp. 15-21, 1935-102X

Solomon, M. J., McLeod, R. S., with the Canadian Task Force on the Periodic Health Examination. (1994). Periodic health examination, 1994 update: 2. Screening strategies for colorectal cancer. *Canadian Medical Association Journal*, Vol. 150, No. 12, (June 1994), pp. 1961-1970, 0820-3946

Strech, D. (2008). Evidence-based ethics—what it should be and what it shouldn't be. *BMC Medical Ethics*, Vol. 9:16, (October 2008), 1472-6939

Sullivan, F. M. & MacNaughton, R. J. (1996). Evidence in consultations: Interpreted and individualized. *Lancet*, Vol. 348, No. 9032, (October 1996), pp. 941-943, 0140-6736

Tallon, D., Chard, J. A., & Dieppe, P. (2000). Relation between agendas of the research community and the research consumer. *Lancet*, Vol. 355, No. 9220, (June 2000), pp. 2037-2040, 0140-6736

Tanenbaum, S. J. (1993). What physicians know. *New England Journal of Medicine*, Vol. 329, No. 17, (October 1993), pp. 1268-1271, 0028-4793

Tanenbaum, S. J. (1994a). Knowing and acting in medical practice: The epistemological politics of outcomes research. *Journal of Health Politics Policy & Law*, Vol. 19, No. 1, (Spring 1994), pp. 27-44, 0361-6878

Tanenbaum, S. J. (1994b). Outcomes research. Author responds. *New England Journal of Medicine*, Vol. 330, No. 6, (February 1994), p. 435, 0028-4793

Tanenbaum, S. J. (1995). Getting from there to here: evidentiary quandaries of the U.S. outcomes movement. *Journal of Evaluation in Clinical Practice*, Vol. 1, No. 2, (November 1995), pp. 97-103, 1365-2753

Upshur, R. E. G., VanDenKerkof, E. G., Goel, V. (2001). Meaning and measure: An inclusive model of evidence in health care. *Journal of Evaluation in Clinical Practice*, Vol. 7, No. 2, (May 2001), pp. 91-96, 1365-2753

Urbach, P. (1993). The value of randomization and control in clinical trials. *Statistics in Medicine*, Vol. 12, No. 15-16, (August 1993), pp. 1421-31, 0277-6715

U.S. Cochrane Center. (2002). *Training Manual for Handsearchers*. In: *Resources for Handsearchers*, October 2011, Available at: http://us.cochrane.org/resources-handsearchers

von Zweck, C. (1999). The promotion of evidence-based occupational therapy practice in Canada. *Canadian Journal of Occupational Therapy*, Vol. 66, No. 5, (December 1999), pp. 208-213, 0008-4174

Wennberg, J. E. (1992). AHCP and the strategy for health care reform. *Health Affairs*, Vol. 11, No. 1, (February 1992), pp. 67-71, 0278-2715

Williams, D. D. R. & Garner, J. (2002). The case against 'the evidence': A different perspective on evidence-based medicine. *British Journal of Psychiatry*, Vol. 180, No. 1, (January 2002), pp. 8-12, 1472-1465

Wood, M., Ferlie, E., & Fitzgerald, L. (1998). Achieving clinical behaviour change: A case of becoming indeterminate. *Social Science and Medicine*, Vol. 47, No. 11, (October 1998), pp. 1729-1758, 02779536

Worrall, J. (2002). What evidence in evidence-based medicine? *Philosophy of Science*, Vol. 69, No. 3, (September 2002), pp. S316-S330, 0031-8248

3

Twenty Lessons to Incorporate EBM Concept and Practices into Medical Education

Madhur Dev Bhattarai
Coordinator Postgraduate Programme of Medicine, Chief, Medical Education Unit, National Academy of Medical Sciences, Bir Hospital, Kathmandu, Nepal

1. Introduction

Evidence-based medicine (EBM) is a new paradigm for the health-care system involving using the current evidence (results of the medical research studies) in the medical literature to provide the best possible care to patients.[1] It has encouraged the rapid and transparent translation of the latest scientific knowledge in the day to day practice of medical professionals. EBM has given new direction in all the fundament responsibilities of medical professionals like care of the patient, research, teaching and learning, and public health. There is need to move from opinion-based education to evidence-based education. Best Evidence Medical Education (BEME) is the implementation of methods and approaches to education based on the best evidence available.[2] The evidence available may be in a wide variety of formats for example: the results of the controlled experimental studies, description of case studies, and opinions of experts. Studies alone are not the evidence.[3] As Hart and Harden have suggested evidence is defined in the American Heritage Dictionary of the English Language as a thing or things helpful in forming a conclusion or judgement.[4,5] The current practices in different regions and institutions in the world will be a form of evidences to consider. Similarly the available evidences in the clinical medicine, or indeed in any other field like airlines industry, need to be correlated with the areas to give focus in the medical education. The text is discussed in four sections, viz. planning of medical education and the community need and service; training and assessment; teachers' criteria and training; and finally individual's mistake, system's error, health safety and trainees. To highlight the key areas of medical education and training requiring attention, the learnings are presented in the form of twenty lessons to consider.

2. Planning of medical education and the community need and service

2.1 Undergraduate medical education

Since seventeen century, different curricular models have been considered which have catalyzed significant changes in the medical education: the apprenticeship model, the discipline-based model, the organ-system-based model, the problem-based-learning model, and the clinical-presentation-based model.[6] These curricula differ to a varying extent in the organization of course content, controllers of content, relationship of clinical to basic sciences, organization of concept formation, teaching methods, timing of patient/case, exposure, cognitive skills emphasized, primary learning guides and problem-solving model.[6] Each has advantages and disadvantages as per the context and mixtures of models are used now in the medical education. In developing countries, the departments in general tend to control the content of the undergraduate medical education as per the discipline-based model, but principles of other models are increasingly being applied.

2.2 Educational strategies

The focus on the undergraduate medical education in the industrialized countries is increasingly on the newer approaches of educational strategy, as opposed to the traditional ones. The newer approaches are highlighted by the SPICES model, consisting of ***S***tudent-centered, ***P***roblem-base, ***I***ntegrated, ***C***ommunity-based, ***E***lectives with a core and ***S***ystematic.[7] These are in contrast to the traditional approaches like ***T***eacher-centered, ***I***nformation gathering, ***D***iscipline-based, ***H***ospital-based, ***U***niform and ***A***pprenticeship. These approaches are self-explanatory, as their names indicate, to some extent and need to be considered and balanced in their spectrums wherever applicable. The problem-based learning approach uses problem-based learning as a vehicle to develop a usable body of integrated knowledge and develop problem-solving skills. A student-centered approach emphasizes on the student, increases motivation and prepares for continuing education.[7] But teachers, students and staff need to adopt and prepare for it. Various approaches depend on the context and situation. However the teaching and learning experiences of students should not be left to chance and it should be planned and recorded and assessed in a systematic manner. Electives allow students to focus as per their need or choice.

2.3 Integrated approach

A number of methods are used to integrate the curriculum, like spiral curriculum and multi-professional learning.[7,8] There is rapid growth of medical colleges in the developing countries leading to dearth of teachers in basic science. A few available basic science teachers may go to different medical colleges and there is tendency of medical colleges even to lure such teachers from other colleges, hampering the teaching of medical students. The acute shortage of basic science teachers in the developing countries has also indirectly raised the need to widen discipline-based approach to integrate the curriculum in the possible ways. The related clinical faculty can undertake the required extra training and then they can be certified for the training of students in the related basic science, for example general surgeons in anatomy, internist in pharmacology, internist and anesthetist in physiology and pathologist in forensic medicine. The teaching by such adjunct clinical faculty will automatically expose the students to the clinical implication of the basic science, making it a sort of applied basic science. The concerned department may be run by the regular faculty and the concerned subject or curriculum committee may be formed by including both the regular and well trained certified adjunct faculties. The regular and the adjunct faculties can learn from each other. The increased interaction will help to develop organ-system-based teaching learning. The exposure and inclusion of the adjunct faculties in the subject committee will also help to arrange early clinical exposure of the students and the vertical integration of the curriculum. In this way, the discipline-based models of the undergraduate medical education will move towards the newer models incorporating the advantages of both discipline-based and integrated approaches.

2.4 Community-based education

In community-based education students are taught in a community setting in contrast to community-oriented education where the focus for teaching is the needs of the community.[8] But in the name of community-based education there may not be much benefit to the student or the community by just posting the students in the community, e.g. for family data collection. The postings of the students covering the overcrowded curriculum should also fulfill the need of the students. If the required and relevant areas, like general practice, internal medicine, pediatric, surgery or obstetrics and gynecology, of the posting for the students are actually practiced in the community, it would be useful to all. For this, the medical institutes should have their own or have affiliation with peripheral institutes providing service to the community in the urban and rural areas. The faculty of the medical institutes can be posted there on rotation and the students will be able to utilize most the posting under their own teacher in the community. It will also directly benefit the community especially in the developing countries, where health-coverage of the general population is inadequate.

2.5 Incorporation of learning theories in the residential training

The learning is not easy to define.[9] The learning theories are also equally, or more complex, to explain. Just knowing something does not complete the definition of learning. From the educational point of view it may broadly be called a process which brings relatively permanent changes in the_way of thinking about and/or feeling about and/or looking at the reality and/or behavior of a learner through experience, education, training, or practice. The change may be temporary or permanent.

The concept about teaching and learning has changed dramatically over the several decades. "Teaching by pouring in" refers to a medieval belief that we teach people by drilling holes in the human head and, with a funnel, pour information into the brain. Then came the era of behaviorism where the issue was not how new knowledge is acquired, but how is new behavior acquired. Behavior can change as a result of extrinsic motivators such as incentives, rewards and punishments, which are utilized in different ways in the training and education in all the fields. Behaviorism is also seen further flourishing with the competency and learning outcomes movement, which focuses exclusively on observable behavior.[10] During the late 1960s and early 1970s cognitivism became popular to understand learning.[10] Cognitivism was closer to a common sense view of how people learned, attempting to map individual thinking processes. The cognitive perspective recognizes the need to build rich, interconnecting knowledge structures, based on existing knowledge, that allows continuing incorporation of new learning. Social cognitive theory (formerly social learning theory) acknowledges the social (interactive) aspect of learning and unites two approaches, behaviorist and cognitive, to understanding knowledge. It posits that our actions, learning and functioning are the result of a continuous, dynamic reciprocal interaction among the three sets of determinants: personal, environmental (situational) and behavioral.[11] Similarly constructivism is based on the premise that the learners construct their own perspective of the world through individual experience and schema.

The ability to reflect on one's practice or performance is critical to lifelong, self-directed learning. At the heart of various learning theories is the belief that we can learn from experience, incorporating it into our existing knowledge and skills. This opportunity for reflection must be actively incorporated and a systematic approach to facilitate reflection must be introduced early. Reflection is not merely description of experience, but analysis of it; it is not a natural and intuitive ability, but must be developed through practice. It is critical to becoming an effective lifelong learner, as it also enables learners to develop and apply standards to their performance, decide what further learning needs to occur, and to continue their learning over a professional lifetime.[11] The concept of the reflective practitioner incorporates all five stages that professionals use in problem solving: knowing-in-action, surprise, reflection-in-action, experimentation, and reflection-on-action. Reflectivity in practice is a learned skill of critical thinking and situational analysis.[11]

Self-directed learning is an aspect of several theoretical approaches, including the cognitive, social learning, humanist and constructivist. Humanist approach views self-direction as evidence of higher level of individual development. Self-directed learning elements can also be seen in the ability to learn from experience, through critical reflection, which allows learners to identify their personal learning needs, and to be aware of, monitor and direct the growth of their knowledge, skills and expertise.[11]

Experiential learning theory considers that learning is best achieved in an environment that considers both concrete experience and conceptual models. There is the necessity of integrating the process of actual experience and education in learning.[11] Learners along the medical educational continuum use various experiential learning methods. These may include: apprentice, internship or practicum, mentoring, clinical supervision, on-the-job training, clinics, case study research.[11] There is a shift away from the older apprenticeship system towards more formal structured training. Structured training focuses on formal skills training, evidence-based accountability, objective evaluation, and competence-based assessment.[12] Old apprenticeship models stressed 'immersion' - the learning by experience simply through exposure. New apprenticeship or 'cognitive apprenticeship' models stress that novices do not simply learn how to 'do' the job as they gain expertise - they also learn how to 'think' and to 'recount' the job.[10] Doing, thinking and recounting are intimately linked as a ground for learning. Medicine is a complex professional practice in which the separation of cognition (thinking), conation (will), affect (feeling), and skill (doing) is impossible and unnecessary and in which individual cognition is secondary to social and other similar effects, i.e. context in learning. Learning implies connections between thinking, sensing, doing, feeling, willing, imagining, intuiting and thinking about thinking (metacognition).[10] After the undergraduate medical education, the medical doctors undergo the structured training programme, commonly called residential training or simply residency, when they work under supervision in the specialty concerned. Most of the theories of learning are incorporated in various forms in the structured residential training at different stages. The focus is on active learning, rather than on passive teaching.[13] Teaching is the process or the 'means' and learning is the outcome or the 'end'. The concept of the structured training programme of residency with actual working in the field under supervision with various teaching-learning and communication activities is to make the learners learn actively and reflectively.

2.6 Continuum of medical education as per the community need

There is continuum of medical education: undergraduate medical education, residential training, and continuing medical education. After undergraduate education, medical doctors have to undergo the structured residential training and accredited appropriately in a specialty before they are allowed to practice. What or where they will practice will depend on the service available in the community. The whole medical education is planned as the need of the community.[14] The service and need of the curriculum decides the medical curriculum. The continuum of medical education and the need of structured training programme of residency are evident by the successful absorption in the US residential programme of thousands of medical graduates taught in different undergraduate curriculums from the developing countries. The structured residential training is obviously important. The undergraduate medical education of whatever curriculum is incomplete without further residential training.

2.7 Lessons learned

Lesson 1: Graduation like MBBS alone not sufficient to allow doctors to practice independently

In the past after graduation the doctors were expected to practice independently with or without having some experience in hospitals. But with increasing vastness of medicine and changing concept of learning and medical education and increasing focus on safety and rights of patients, such independent practice for any medical graduate is not possible now in the industrialized countries. Many lessons could also be learnt from the evidences of the background and implementations of series of health and educational reports and reforms, like Tomorrow's Doctors, Modernizing Medical Careers and others in different parts of the world.[15-18] With the rapid and massive growth of diagnostic and therapeutic interventions and specializations, the need of structured residency programmes for medical training is more now. Without even the basic training of the medical profession of vast majority of medical doctors, it will be difficult, if not impossible, to implement evidence-based medicine. Thus every medical graduate now needs to undertake structured-residential training to practice clinical medicine.

Lesson 2: Structured training programme of residency is a 'must' in postgraduate medical education

As discussed above, after graduation, medical professionals need to undergo supervised, structured residential training of actual working to fulfill the required evidences to be fit to practice in any field. In developing countries, many postgraduate degrees are awarded without residential programme. Evidences are clear that such 'theoretical' or 'library' degrees, either for national or foreign students, are not valid for any clinical practice on human beings. Training and learning would not be acquired without working as residents. Teaching and learning basically occur while managing cases in the units. The focus is on developing skills of reflexivity, not just remembering. The residents have to manage patients and face different situations, so the materials to be learned are personally relevant and responsibilities to learn fall on the learners themselves as well. This is an example of task-based learning, the strategy that focuses student learning around real cases that the students meet in the wards, out-patient departments and emergency.[19] The meaningfully learned knowledge is retrievable, durable and generalisable. The students acquire basic science knowledge and clinical reasoning skills in the context of actual patient care.[11]

Lesson 3: The candidates selection for any Sub-Specialist Training should only be from among those who have already completed General Specialist Training

After the undergraduate medical education, for clinical practice every graduate will have to undergo General (or Basic) Specialist Training. After the General Specialist Training, they can join the medical practice in the relevant subject or can continue Sub- (or Higher-) Specialist Training.[16-18] The general outline of the training of the medical professionals is shown in the Figure 1.

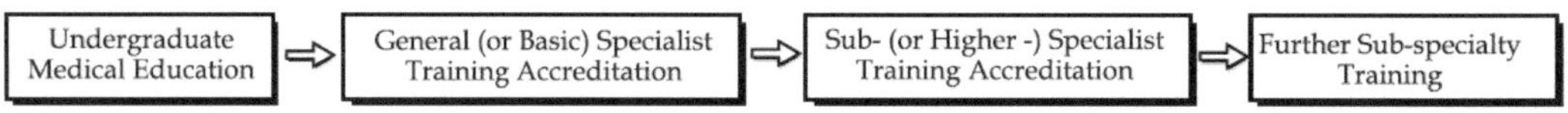

Fig. 1. The continuum of education of the medical professionals: The medical graduate can only practice in any specialty after the necessary accreditation in the relevant field after undergoing structured-residential training.

After graduation, medical professionals need to undergo supervised, structured residential training of actual working and get accredited in the General Specialty like General Surgery, Internal Medicine, General Practice or others. Then they can either practice in the General Specialty or go for Sub-Specialist Training similarly in different sub-specialties like cardiology, diabetes, urology and others.[16-18] Each step of requirement is important to go to the next phase. The 'experience of working' alone in any basic specialties, medicine or surgery, will not fulfill the requirement to allow the candidates go to higher specialties, like gastroenterology or urology, training. But direct enrolment and teaching in different sub-specialities is practiced in many 'postgraduate' programmes in the developing countries. The candidates for any Sub-Specialist Training should not be enrolled before they complete the relevant General Specialist Training. Similarly the experts need to consider whether direct orthopedic training, as practiced in many countries, should be allowed or not without first undergoing the training in General Surgery, particularly if the orthopedicians primarily manage trauma patients, and trauma units or centers.

Lesson 4: Need of structured residential training programme in General Practice

Evidences are clear that medical professionals need to fulfill the required evidences to be fit to practice in any field before they can be allowed to practice independently. Similar requirements are required for anyone to practice as Generalist in rural or urban areas. General Practitioners have to manage from medicine to surgery, pediatric to geriatric, orthopedics to obstetrics, and other. Residential training in General Practice provides the necessary medical professionals to serve in the community as practiced in industrialized as well as now in some developing countries in the world.[16-18,20] Similar program is required in other countries before the medical graduates can practice in the rural or urban community. Such practitioners will also be the most appropriate personnel to be further trained for some months in health administration or public health to take such responsibilities later; this would also provide them further career incentive.

Lesson 5: Need of structured training programme, with appropriate eligibility criteria, in infectious diseases

Communicable or infectious diseases are major public health burdens in the developing countries.[21] But there is scarcity of Sub-Specialist Training programmes in Infectious Diseases for the medical professionals already qualified with General-Specialist Training in Internal Medicine to produce infectious disease specialists.[20,22,23] That could be one of major reasons of not having adequate service and data of infectious diseases in the developing countries. The trend now is to train the medical professionals in the Infectious Diseases after the General Specialist Training programme of residency in Internal Medicine.[16-18] Similar program is required in the developing countries to produce appropriate consultants and leaders in this common major problem of infectious diseases, including HIV/AIDS, tuberculosis, hepatitis and others.

Lesson 6: Need of appropriate eligibility criteria for the educational course of public health and health-service administration

Health administration plans and mobilizes the health professional service in any country. The service decides the curriculum for the training of health professionals in any community.[14] So health-service administration is a key point and personnel need to have experience and concepts of both the medical education and health problems in the community. Medical doctors just with the undergraduate education, like MBBS, may not have full concepts of the health problems even with any other administrative training alone. Similarly in the public health, training the MBBS, or non-MBBS, graduates only with some months of master in public health training program may not now produce appropriate experienced professionals to give the required leadership in this vital field. The varied eligibility criteria for such course in public health seems to be creating confusion in the hierarchy of postings and in the planning and implementation of the necessary programmes in the developing countries. General Practitioners or other practitioners who have had undergone structured training programme after medical graduation may be the appropriate personals to be further trained in health administration or public health for some months to take such responsibilities. This would also be a career incentive for General Practitioners in the rural and urban community. Thus the training programme in public health and health-service administration needs to be discussed and planned considering the implications and the contexts.

Lesson 7: Public health institutes have to be involved in the structured training or postgraduate programmes

The opportunity for structured training in the developing countries is severely limited by the concept of giving 'postgraduate degrees' mostly inside the closed-wall of medical colleges,[20,22] which are increasingly becoming private and charge exorbitant fees. The mass of people in developing countries attend public institutes, which are not given the due priority, or even attention, for improvement in the quality, as if EBM is only to be taught by the professors in the medical colleges. Whereas the public health institutes itself could also be easily included in the structured training of medical graduates improving the quality of the public health institutes and increasing the training venues to adequately train the medical graduates efficiently, as evident in the industrialized, as well as in some developing, countries.[16-18,24,25] If the quality of the public hospitals is not taken care of, the situation of the private institutions could become even worse. Considering the rapid and massive growth of diagnostic and therapeutic interventions and specializations, it may not be possible to keep all the facilities for patient care and residents' training under one roof or closed-wall of a medical institute, especially for the Sub-Specialist Training. Demographic and environmental conditions may also lead to variation in the types and cases of patients visiting any particular institute. Apart from the private medical colleges, other private medical institutes may also be included in the training programme if the facilities and patients are available. As the teaching-learning is a part of professionalism of medical professionals, the consultants and other specialists can easily be trained to be a supervisor and faculty for the training programme. The university and medical colleges can affiliate with the public hospitals for teaching-learning and service activities and can also develop their own medical centers in the peripheral part of the country. The students and the faculty of the medical institutes can be posted there on rotation in their required specialties in the peripheral health centers, which will also help the undergraduates and residents to get the experience of community-based education (as discussed in 2.4).

Lesson 8: Residential training, as well as later revalidation and appraisal, programmes are the responsibilities of the State, not of individual medical institutes or trainees

The structured residential postgraduate programmes need to be planned and supervised by the State as in the industrialized countries.[16-18] Committee or councils are required to accredit institutes, like medical schools and public and private institutes, for training and similarly to accredit the structured residential programme.[16-18] Subdivisions of the required functions for the training and registration of medical professionals and their relation with different institutes where structured training programme could be arranged are shown in the Figure 2. Relevant experts from different fields can be the members of the committees. There can be overlap of representatives from different stakeholders in the committees as per the local situation. But the academic requirements and programmes need to be guided by the principles and committees of the State. Registration of medical practitioners by the State is in general a separate issue (Figure 2). Identification and regulation of separate functions helps to promote their appropriate planning and implementation. But in many countries, all

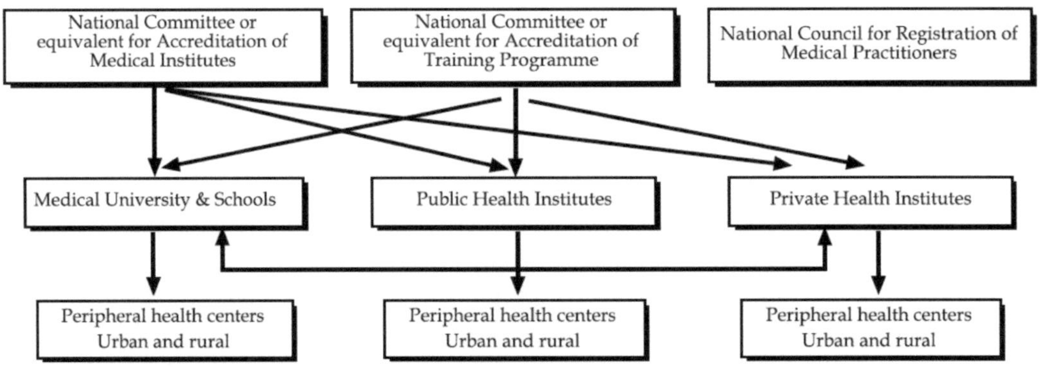
National Committee or equivalent for Accreditation of Medical Institutes
National Committee or equivalent for Accreditation of Training Programme
National Council for Registration of Medical Practitioners
Medical University & Schools
Public Health Institutes
Private Health Institutes
Peripheral health centers Urban and rural
Peripheral health centers Urban and rural
Peripheral health centers Urban and rural

Fig. 2. Subdivisions of the required functions for the training and registration of medical professionals and their relation with different institutes where structured training programme could be arranged: There can be overlap of representatives from different stakeholders in the committees.

the three functions are managed by medical council.[20,22] It would not be easy for any single organization to plan and manage different types of the functions requiring different approaches appropriately, which may, not surprisingly, lead to inefficiency and even corruption often heard in the developing countries. In UK, before the Calman reforms trainees were expected to organize their own training programmes. After the introduction of reforms the control and responsibility for the organization of training shifted to the committees.[26] Structured residential training, as well as later revalidation and appraisal, programmes are the responsibilities of the State for the safety and health of the people.

Lesson 9: Training of the medical professionals is planned as per the community need

Medical education and curriculum is guided by the community situation, practice and need.[14] Community need may change as per the population demographics, disease patterns, resources and possible services. Specialty and subspecialty service development would be as per the local situation including volume of patients to justify the separate service, time of the available experts and the duration of training required to develop the expertise. The medical service practice in the community based on the available human resources may need to be restructured later differently for the effective and safe service delivery to the people considering the changing situation and teaching and learning concepts, increasing human resources and population as well as demand of the people, and trends in other parts of the world. For example, in many developing countries the patients in the emergency and observation wards are often managed by other speciality units, including Internal Medicine units, of the hospital and in this situation emergency department, simply a patient-entry point venue for other specialties to manage the patient, is easily coordinated by the General Pracititioners even without any extra training. If the Emergency or Acute Medicine is to be practiced independently as in many industrialized countries, then internists may need to be further trained for it. Similarly, the intensive care or treatment units (ICU/ITU), especially the ventilatory and other related aspects, in the developing countries are managed, along with other related units, usually by the anesthetists or by respiratory physicians now in some places. But the Critical Care Medicine is itself becoming a separate sub-specialty service and training area from the Internal Medicine stream. With increasing number of elderly population the need of Geriatric Medicine service and training is also obvious. Thus, the training courses for different higher specialties practice are guided by the community service need. The community need may be different in affluent or non-affluent and sparse or densely populated areas even in the same country whether industrialized or developing one. Some possible service, career and training options of Internal Medicine, General Practice and General Surgery and their sub-specialties in the community are shown in Figures 3, 4 and 5 respectively. For the situation of the scarce human resources or patient-loads, like in rural areas, the trainees from the general stream of General Practice could be given extra required training in obstetrics and gynaecology and anesthesia to practice as rural general practitioner (Figure 4). There will be similar options of services and trainings for other specialties like Paediatrics, Obstetrics and Gynaecology, Radiology, Pathology and others. After the General Specialist Training in any specialties, a faculty can be fully trained in Medical (Health Professional) Education specialty. The proportions of the numbers of the training opportunities for General Practice and other General and Sub-Specialty Trainings should be decided as per the requirements of the community and the later possible careers. Whether the Dental Surgeons should first undergo general medical undergraduate education followed by General Specialist Training in Dental field is a matter which can be discussed by the relevant experts, especially for the overlapping fields like oral-maxillary-facial surgery.[27]

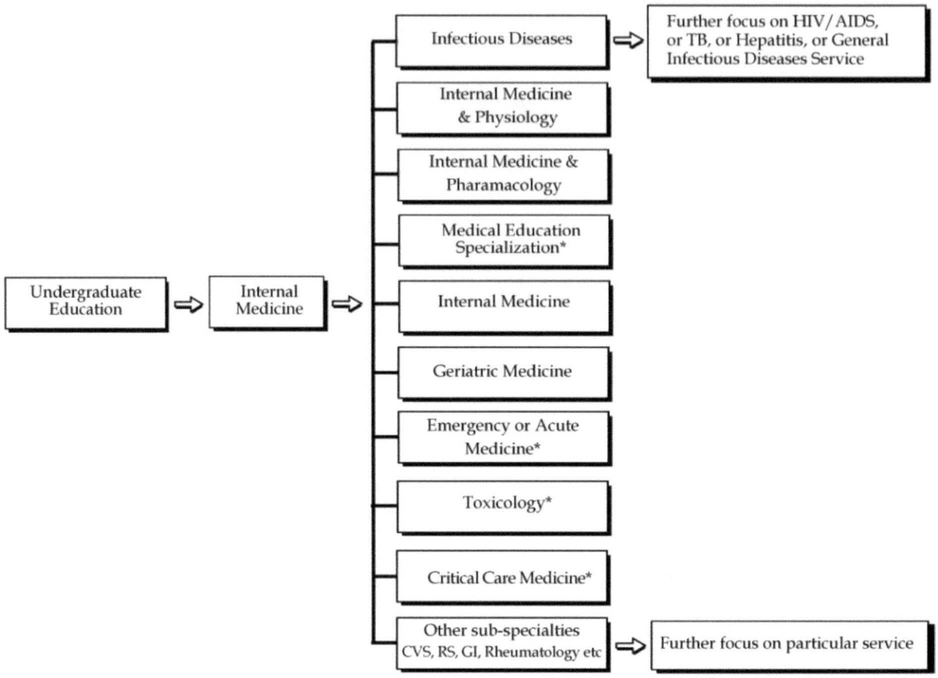

*The extra service can be continued along with the Internal Medicine as per the volume of workload, time of the available experts and training required in the subject.

Fig. 3. Some possible options of services of Internal Medicine and its sub-specialties in the community, according to which the training of the medical professionals need to be arranged.

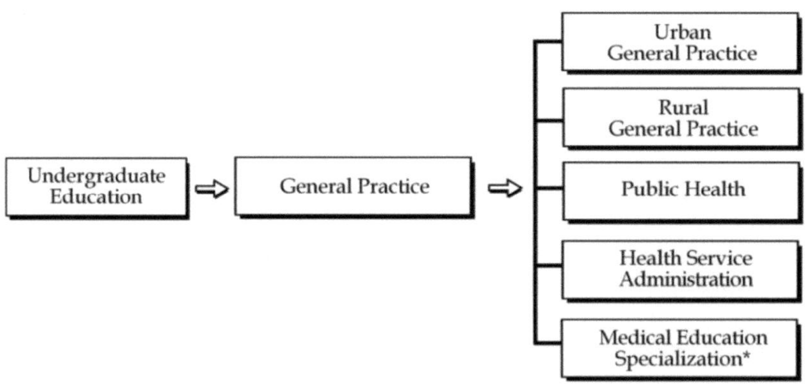

*The extra service an be continued along with the General Practice as per the volume of workload, time of the available experts and training required in the subject.

Fig. 4. Some possible options of services of General Practice and its sub-specialties in the community, according to which the training of the medical professionals need to be arranged.

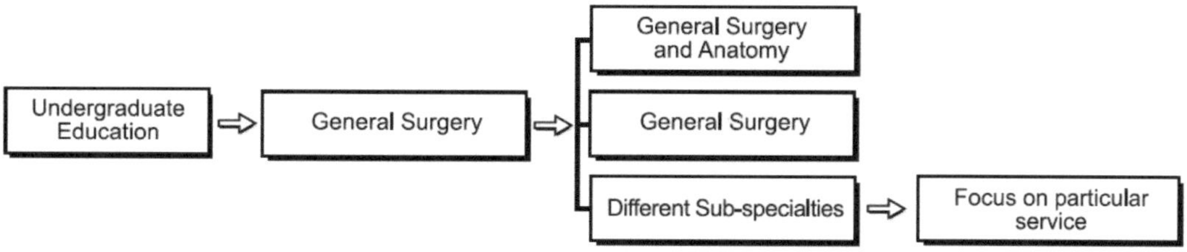

Fig. 5. Some possible options of services of General Surgery and its sub-specialties in the community, according to which the training of the medical professionals need to be arranged.

Lesson 10: Structured-residential programme involves doing the required work entitling the full pay and continuation of the service without any extra-training fee

Every medical graduate needs to undergo residential training before they can serve as a medical professional.[15-18] Even while they are undergoing structured-training programme, they are working in the field of their career and serving the community. Thus residential programme, whether General Specialist or Sub-Specialist Training, is like in-service training, not requiring any special leave or extra-payment for the training. During the residential training, the residents provide efficient and actual service to the people for which they should be paid as well as such residential training, unlike undergraduate medical or other non-residential non-service providing higher education, should be free not requiring any extra-training fee as in many industrialized countries. This is different from educational programmes of other service personnel in any institute or national service, where people may have to take special leave to study without doing their assigned jobs. The medical training and service are interrelated. The formal inclusion of the concept will help the career and morale of the trainees which is important for the better service and care of the patients. The trainees can thus continue their sub-specialty training as per their choice and service.

3. Training and assessment

Optimal training of the residents is a key concern of all the stakeholders. The focus of teachers and curriculum planners is to provide appropriate training. But active participation of the learners is required. Students may not realize and give full attention to the concept of the training. Passing the examination is the major focus of students. Students naturally tailor their learning styles to the assessment demands. They are very quick to respond to what they perceive as the demands of the assessment system.[28] The content of the assessment will become in reality the course objective. For example, if it becomes widely known that topic 'A' is never included in any examination, it is difficult, if not impossible, to persuade students that mastery of it should be an objective for their studies.[28] Thus, assessment methods and criteria are the most effective tools we have to help all students achieve training criteria and ultimately pass. The curriculum planner and faculty need to understand the relation between the training and assessment criteria (Figure 6), and especially the fact that assessment is basically for training, not just for certification. The educational impact of the assessment on the learning of students is significant and faculty must utilize it to the maximum.

"It is the examination system rather than educational objectives, curriculum organization, or educational techniques that had the most profound impact upon student learning. For no matter

how appealing the statement of goals, how logical the program organization, how dazzling the teaching methods, it is the examination that communicated most vividly to students what was expected of them"

--George E Miller

"Students work to pass, not to know......They do pass and they don't know"

--Thomas Huxley

"Learning, teaching and assessment must not be viewed as isolated concepts. In the ideal scenario effective teaching, effective learning and effective assessment are all part of the same educational process. The value of changing assessment to reflect what needs to be learned is evident since students learn what they will be tested on"

--Doyle, 1983

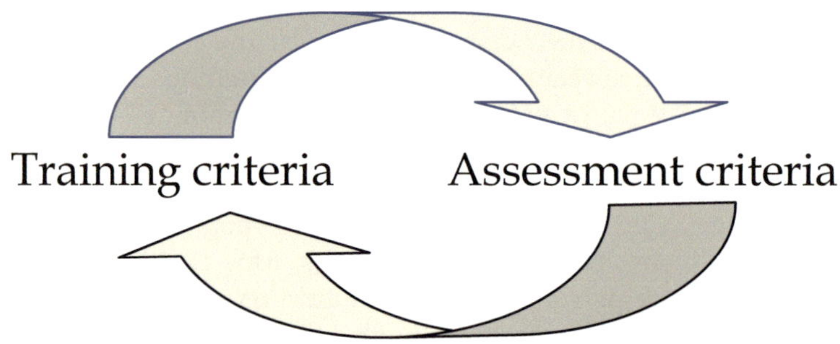

Fig. 6. The close relation between training and assessment criteria.

The assessment criteria should be clearly spelled out as per the outcomes we want of the products of the training. While preparing the assessment criteria, the faculty need to consider the training need of the students for the specialty in the local community and such criteria then should be made known to the students, so that they try to prepare accordingly, which in the process helps them to achieve the expected training need. We can, thus, say: "Whatever you want your students to do, include it as a part of the assessment first, and then only they will learn and do actively!"

3.1 Criterion-referenced assessment

The principal objective of medical education is to produce a competent physician. Unquestionably, the basic aim and approach for the evaluation process is to assess the standard of competency and not the rank order of students.[29] The assessment which simply ranks the order of performance in terms of their position in the group is norm- or normative-referenced assessment. The norm-referenced assessment fails to providea clear picture of what the student can or cannot do. It does not provide useful feedback i.e. pinpoint strengths and weakness and it cannot discern to what degree an educational programme has met these standards.[29] Recognising the norm-referenced assessment's limitations, Glasser in 1963 formalised the concept of criterion-referenced assessment.[30] Standards of performance are set using minimal levels of competence before the test is applied. The assessor sets the level of performance which is required. It may be the total mastery of a task or it may be the minimal acceptable level. The criteria-referenced assessment allows pinpointing students' capabilities i.e. what they can or cannot do. Thus criterion-referenced testing must become the principal method of evaluation within medical education. "Meeting the required standards" and "Fitness for purpose" are two notions that highlight quality assurance.[31] Both are related ideas in that we need to consider the criteria against which the achievement of standards is going to be measured, and a major criterion must surely be the fitness for purpose. This certification cannot be achieved just by the theory or clinical practical examination in the exit examination. A mixture of assessment criteria and methods has to be documented.

3.2 Exit examination and the eligibility criteria for the exit examination

Apart from the assessment in the exit examination, the eligibility for the exit examination has to be defined by the criteria to be fulfilled. Once eligibility is expressed clearly, then it is obvious that all candidates have to achieve it before they can appear in exit examination and subject committees and examination section have to ensure they are achieved. Passing the examination is the major focus of students. Indeed, regulations, like the eligibility for final exit examination, and examination are the only 'languages' students try to understand fully and take seriously. Each component and criterion of the examination is vital to train the students appropriately and needs serious attention.

3.3 Lessons learned

Lesson 11: Spell out the eligibility criteria for the exit examination

The eligibility criteria for the exit examination will vary as per the level of assessment, situation of the service and need in the community where the candidates will later work, and the specialty. There is a example of ten criteria of assessment for the exit examination of residential-programme in the General Specialist Training.[32] In general, the outline of the possible eligibility criteria for the exit examination could be considered in the following headings:

- Adequate attendance of actual working as a resident with regular and emergency duties
- Achievement of the minimum pass-percentage in the required theory and clinical examination held earlier
- Completion of horizontal and vertical, i.e. spiral upward, rotation training posting
- Completion of minimum numbers of most important, e.g. top 10, procedures and/or experiences
- Completion of relevant mandatory basic courses, like advanced cardiac life support (ACLS), communication skills including breaking bad news, learning principles and methods, evidence-based medicine, basic surgical skills, trauma-life support, palliative care, and others
- Completion of portfolio focused on communication
- Completion of minimum numbers of presentations, e.g. journal, case, topic and others
- Completion of minimum numbers of teaching to juniors and nurses

Lesson 12: Assess the required basic theory and clinical components in the early part of the training programme

One of the characteristics of the adult learners is that they base their learning upon the experiences they have.[33] The skills required for patient care depend upon learning in both the theory and clinical areas.[13] A lack of solid base of knowledge foundation, including applied basic science, during the clinical training programme will be a serious handicap for learning the concepts of the subject. If the students can correlate and apply their knowledge to the patient care related to the subject of postgraduation during the context of their training, then they are likely to have the full understanding of the concepts and principles of the specialty. For this purpose, the students have to acquire the required base of knowledge on time during the initial phase of training itself. The students give priority to the assessment. If the theory examination, including of the applied basic science, is held at the end of the final year, the students will naturally prepare for it at that time only. But the aim is not just to assess knowledge of the students at the end, but to train them in their actual field of specialization integrating all the required knowledge. Thus the basic or minimum theory and clinical components required for the training to be assessed in the early part of the training-programme have to be decided and arranged in the required scheduled. The training and assessment have to be primarily managed by the faculty of the relevant specialty, not by the basice science teachers. Such assessment would help to achieve the aim of formative assessment, which is the identification of deficiency during the training period in order to correct them. The possible topics, areas and questions to be asked in such assessment may be published as a guidebook and given to the students, so that they can prepare themselves for the examination. The role of study guides in facilitating and managing independent learning is well accepted.[34]

Lesson 13: Plan appropriately the horizontal and vertical, i.e. spiral upward, rotation training posting

In postgraduate residential training, the students are rotated in different units related to their subject of post-graduation. During such rotations, the training and exposure in different sub-specialties required and the sufficient work load and other learning opportunities available should be considered to decide regarding the postings and their durations. The specialties for the residents to be rotated need to be correlated with the actual responsibilities they will be fulfilling later after the training. For example, in Internal Medicine rotation in psychiatry, diabetes, infectious diseases, ICU/ITU and CCU may be equally, if not more, relevant that in gastroenterology and cardiology alone if the residents later are not going to do any invasive or non-invasive procedures of gastroenterology and cardiology. For this, the subject committee may have to consider the types of patients managed by the general medicine unit and decide as per the local context. The postings planned a few years back will have to be reviewed as per the changing situation. The other important point to consider is that the training during the rotation postings is not just horizontal; it is also vertical and progressive,i.e. spiral upward. In the beginning of the training, the students are posted as junior residents in their subject of post-graduation for about some months to a year to get the basic knowledge and skills. Next they will be rotated in different subspecialties or related units as rotating residents. Finally they need to be rotated back as senior residents to their subject of post-graduation for about a year to assimilate or integrate all the learning. During this final posting as senior residents, they work with increased experience and responsibility of managing the unit with wider perspective and decision making responsibility, including supervision of junior residents, thus, to have the overview of the subject. The concept of problem based learning (PBL), i.e. a learning strategy characterized by self-directed active learning starting with problems or inquiries that learners themselves identify[35] is thus inherently incorporated in the third year posting. It is well said that a good surgeon knows how to operate, a better surgeon knows when to operate and the best surgeon knows when not to operate. The decision making training in the specialty to be certified can be given in the final phase of posting in that subject. Approximately 75% of the significant events in surgical procedure are linked to decision making and about 25% to manual skills.[36] Thus appropriate horizontal and vertical rotation training postings need to be planned.

Lesson 14: Spell out the minimum numbers of most important, e.g. top 10, procedures and/or experiences

Postgraduate residents are required to maintain a record (log) book of the work carried out by them.[20,22,23] But without the specifications of the minimum numbers of experiences required, checking the logbook with details of the entries of so manjy procedures and activities will just make it a formality for the residents to get it signed, even at the last hour before examination. If the minimum number of the top ten procedures or experience is spelled out, the verification of their completion by the subject committee can then be easily made as one of the eligibility criteria to be fulfilled before the final exit examination.[24,25,32] The spelling out the minimal number of most important procedures and/or experience in the curriculum and logbook will automatically ensure fulfillment of many other necessary background experience as well.[32] The principle objective of structured residential training programme is to produce a competent specialist. At the end of the training programme, it is necessary to certify the candidate's level of knowledge, skill and competence. The clear specification of operative skills is particularly vital in surgical specialties. For example to certify a medical profession as a trained in General Surgery, it has to be assured that the candidate has the necessary experience of working in General Surgery and s/he has achieved the necessary competency level to operate the required surgeries like appendicectomy or cholecystectomy independently etc. With the documentation of such criteria of important procedures, then external examiners and reviewers can also give necessary feedback. The experts in the field may also need to discuss the related vital issues, for example "What is the domain of General Surgery now in the changing medical and demographic scenario like increasing old age and problem of benign prostatic hypertrophy, development of laprascopic surgery, the scarcity of urology operation theatre (OT) and redundancy of general surgical service with mostly asymptomatic gall stones available to fill the OT list?"; or "Should the senior faculty and consultants in the General Surgeon Unit perform transurethral resection of prostate with Urologists dealing the area beyond the prostate?" and others.[37]

Lesson 15: Need of skill laboratory for the safe and appropriate training of the residents

The rapid expansion of medical knowledge and medical procedures, lesser working hours available and longer years of training required considering the learning curve for appropriate competency and patient safety indicate the value and need of skill lab in clinical and procedural training. Simulation-based medical education is now recognized as an increasingly powerful complementary teaching methodology in the medical profession. It is driven by a combination of the forces; they are: the patient safety movement, objective structured clinical examinations, patient rights movements and patient ethical issues, animal rights movements, risk management and medicolegal atmosphere, economic forces, and the simulation industry.[38] Experienced surgeons, if they desire to learn an innovative procedure, students and surgical trainees have to pass through a learning curve to acquire any particular new skills. This learning curve is usually constructed in retrospect, rather than being applied as a continuous assessment based on predetermined criteria. It is possible to predict the extent of a learning curve.[39] For example, Yaegashi et al relied upon operating time and blood loss when suggesting that gynecology trainees need to perform more than 75 hysterectomies to achieve competence in the procedure.[40] Surgeons can become proficient after performing about 25 laparoscopic antireflux procedures.[41,42] It would be ideal if the learning curve for all the surgical procedures could be measured. Learning by 'service saturation' has to change in response to the decrease in hours that surgical trainees can work.[39] Thus it is increasingly crucial to take advantage of the educational value of every experience in an effort to shorten the length of the learning curve for new procedures. Teaching and development of practical skills is now frequently done in workshops and skills laboratories. It requires specialist materials and equipment, smaller class size and longer blocks of time for practice.[39] The use of simulation has the potential to allow measurement of performance and establish objective metrics that can be used for formative and summative assessments. This is of crucial importance if we are to consider the development of proficiency-based curricula rather than time-based educational programs. Different kinds of tools to teach practical skills are available like printed materials, mannekin, video, multimedia, complex manipulation simulators, integrated procedure simulators, laprascopic simple box trainers, virtual laparoscopic trainers, and others.[39] Virtually reality technology have been used widely in aviation training and more recently it has been adapted for use in surgery.[39] A virtual reality simulator can offer the chance for the learner to repeatedly practice a manual skill until it is technically perfected. To utilize the resources effectively, especially if scarce, the skill lab can be developed with mutual collaboration as a common training venue for trainees from different institutes. International agencies and the institutes of industrialized countries should come forward to help establishing the skill lab in developing countries. Indeed the institutes in the industrialized countries can also be benefited by the mutual collaboration. Low resource centers may have volumes of patients and procedures and other varieties of disease patterns useful for the appropriate trainees from abroad. Thus both can benefit from cooperation, including faculty exchange and discussion forums. The experts from industrialized countries can visit low resource centers to help setting-up newer diagnostic and therapeutic modalities and units.

Lesson 16: The thesis-study not appropriate now for the residential training programme

Submission and approval of thesis work is a well known pre-requisite to become eligible to appear in the final exit examination in postgraduate clinical training programme in the developing countries.[20,22,23] But in the changing situation of present context it appears to be a high-time to consider whether we should continue to keep thesis study as the necessary component in the clinical residential training of medical professionals. There is a rapid and massive growth of diagnostic and therapeutic interventions and specializations. It could be difficult for the residents to cope with the training and learning requirements related to their own field and thesis-study on human subjects, including children and pregnant women, could hamper the actual training required. Moreover the requirements required to conduct research in humans are clear and established now. Medical professionals need separate training and certification for conducting research. Both students and their guides, with burdens of and primary focus on service and teaching responsibilities, may not have enough time for or may not be well trained to conduct research mostly on patients attending health institutes only for seeking treatment. The residents are students in the phase of learning of their own field, even leaving aside the research principles. The clinical training itself is getting more complex with rapid growth in technology, globalization and increasing expectation of the population. The structured residential training is required for all medical graduates. With the increasing number of trainees it could be more difficult, if not impossible, for the institutional review boards and research councils to make adequate supervision of such studies in the developing countries with likelihood of harms to the patients. It is, thus, an issue of basic safety and rights of the patients in the developing countries where illiteracy and ignorance of rights are also high. Conducting thesis-study is not necessary to learn EBM. EBM could be learned by mandatory basic course training on EBM, journal club, applying EBM in each patient and learning the development of one's practicing field. Requirement of thesis-study is not there in the clinical training programmes of many industrialized countries.[16-18] If the thesis-study is not required, the number of residents to be enrolled to structured training programme of residency will also not be limited by the availability of faculty who can fulfill the criteria to guide the thesis work. The residents for the structured-training programme could, then, be admitted or enrolled as per the required training possible in the specialty under the supervision of the senior faculties who are already as such managing the unit and providing the necessary service to the community.

Lesson 17: Assessment of history taking, physical examination and communication is necessary in the exit examination of residential training programme

All evidences point the importance of history and communication in the patient management. Current evidence suggest that most diagnoses result from findings in the history, and to a lesser extent, the physical examination and laboratory testing.[43,44] Similarly, failures in communication are the most frequent source of patient dissatisfaction. Some 70% of lawsuits are a result of poor communication rather than failures of biomedical practice.[45] Thus adequate training of communication and history taking is obviously important. Training and assessment of communication, including history taking, done during the undergraduate education before the beginning of the structured-residential training alone will not be sufficient. Effective history taking and communication depends on the base knowledge, experience of actual working in the specialty, and the practice of doing so during the residential training. If there is no assessment of the history taking and communication in the training programme of the residency, the students may not give much attention to it and may not try to gain knowledge about it or adopt practice. But the training assessments may be focused just on multiple-choice questions (MCQs) considering its reliability.[16,17] An instrument may be perfectly reliable but totally invalid. For example, an MCQ examination may show high reliability but is it really a valid measure of whether students are competent in resuscitation skills or history taking and communication?[47] Existing methods of assessment of history taking and communication, e.g. modified OSCEs, multiple long cases, observed long cases, videos, simulated/standardized patients and others, may not have that high reliability. But that does not mean a method just because of its high reliability can replace a valid method of assessment especially when evidences are clear that value of communication is high in diagnosis as well as patient satisfaction and reducing medical error. In the criterion-referenced assessment, like for the accreditation of medical professional, validity is the priority to give attention particularly when the assessment is considered along with a mixture of criteria. Whereas in the normative-referenced assessment, like in entrance examination for any programme or job, reliability assumes more importance than validity to remove any selection bias, or even possibility of nepotism or corruption (Figure 7). From this point of view reliability appears to support rights of the students and validity appears to support rights (and safety) of the patients. Using and finding reliable ways to make the valid assessment would be preferred in criterion-referenced assessment than using reliable method of assessment which is less valid.

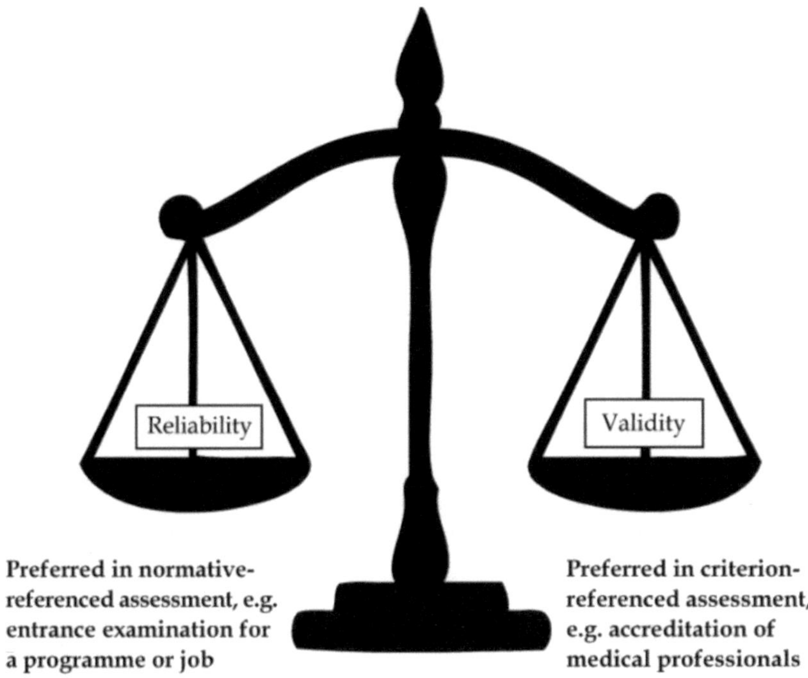

Fig. 7. Balancing reliability and validity as the assessment tool

Lesson 18: Include training in communication and reflection in the General Specialist Training programme

Different methods of teaching like case-based discussion, feedback, directly observed history taking, clinical examination and procedure performance are increasingly included now in the residential training. Many of these aspects can be efficiently incorporated in the ambulatory care setting of outdoor clinics by quick methods of teaching like one-minute preceptor model. Training programmes, most importantly, also need to be planned directly to cover communication, including breaking bad news and communication in consultation, by the communication and medical education experts. Communication training during undergraduate medical education without the required base knowledge of the subject of specialization and regular exposure during the residential training will not be enough for the requirements during the residential training. The communication is a daily, almost continuous, affair in the medical world. Valuable learning can be acquired from any experience in the medical training by reflection and further learning efforts.[11] For this, apart from the other face-to-face training programs on communication, the learning-portfolio in the field of communication is of immense help.[48-51] Repeated training of all the residents is not feasible, but portfolio on communication gives an opportunity to learn from every encounter of communication. Learning-portfolio also helps the residents to develop the quality of reflective practitioner. Reflection is an essential component for the development of a learning cycle and life-long learning required for the professionals. It is essential for medical professionals to continue their personal learning plans as per the different developments and requirements later in their career. The accreditation process of the specialists should of course depend on fulfilment of work-designated responsibilities and requirements, not just on achievement of personal learning plans. Learning-portfolio is one of the useful approaches to facilitate reflection.[49-51] Thus, portfolio focused on communication would help the residents to improve their communication as well as the habit of reflection.

4. Teachers' criteria and training

The twelve roles of the teacher are well known: clinical or practical teacher and lecturer as information provider, on-the-job role model and teaching role model as medical expertise, learning facilitator and mentor as facilitator, student assessor and curriculum evaluator as assessor, curriculum planner and course organizer as planner, and study guide producer and resource material creator as resource developer.[52] For the General or Sub-Specialty training of the residents the most important roles expected from the vast majority of faculty are those of medical expertise and supervision. They can then be easily trained in other common responsibilities regularly required for all viz. learning-facilitator and students-assessment. Some can be trained to coordinate development of resource and organization of course. A few will need to focus on curriculum planning and curriculum evaluation. The point to note is that in the twelve roles of the teachers, conducting studies and publication of paper on clinical aspects are as such not emphasized. But in the teachers criteria the focus is only in paper publication in their fields in many parts of the world.[20,22,23] The teaching faculty designations itself appears to be linked more with the ideas of any research and paper publication, rather than with educational activities.[20,22] Due to the minimum criteria required of the teachers to have done thesis-study previously and publish number of original articles, there is scarcity of teachers, when the need of today is to provide the opportunity of residential training to 'all' medical graduates, not just a few ones. The residents for the structured-training programme should be admitted or enrolled as per the required and relevant work available in the specialty, for which they are being trained. Thus there is dire need to consider appropriately the definition of the domains of the teachers and the criteria required for them which are separate from those of other academic positions. The teaching responsibility of the medical professionals deserves appropriate attention, priority, and 'glamorization' equal to, if not more than, their role as researcher.[32]

4.1 Lesson learned

Lesson 19: Make appropriate teachers' criteria and plan necessary training accordingly

The teachers' criteria for the residential training programme should be based on the most important role expected from the vast majority of faculty, which is clinical and practical and patient management skills. Any faculty or consultant are likely to have such expertize required for that contexts. Subsequently teachers' training needs to be planned and other requirements to be laid down to continue as teachers. Shorter overview training covering the spectrums of teaching-learning activities, lesson-planning, class-room teaching and communication skills, feedback method, ambulatory teacher-learning, assessment and other similar ones may be required for all. Specific workshops and training will be useful for assessment methods, microteaching, lesson-planning and other skills. Constructive feedback is an essential responsibility of all teachers for which they should be trained.[54] As the focus of healthcare provision shifts towards ambulatory care, increasing attention must now be given to developing opportunities for clinical teaching in this setting.[55] Many specialties like dermatology, ophthalmology, general practice, diabetes and others have significant ambulatory service. The number of residents in such specialties will not be dependent on the indoor works and bed numbers, but will depend on workload and opportunities for learning in the ambulatory care settings. Support and training of teachers and supervisors is essential in improving the quality of postgraduate medical education. All faculties may not have the similar roles. After the initial general training of the junior faculty, portfolio on postgraduate training will be useful to remind them regularly the various aspects of teaching-learning.[56] The portfolio can be for learning or assessment.[49-51] Audit, including of teaching-learning activities, will also be useful for junior faculty. The value of audit is well established and popular in industrialized countries since more than two decades in improving patient care as part of an ongoing educational process, basically involving change management and quality assurance.[57,58] Training on preparation of study guides will be useful for majority. The role of study guides in facilitating and managing independent learning is well accepted.[34] The requirements of research training certification and paper publications, including on medical education, will also be applicable to the various academic faculty positions, especially the senior ones, but this should not prevent the enrolment of the medical graduates for the structured residential training. The criteria for teachers for residential training is a separate issue than that for other academic faculty positions. Thus the teachers' criteria, benefits and training need to match the expected training of the residents and provide the opportunities for training for all the medical graduates in the community.[32] The faculty position designations of the teachers may be categorized based on different educational activities, involvement or roles like on-the-job training and supervision, clinical teaching, small group facilitation, assessment, curriculum management and planning, mentoring, audit, portfolio, study guide development, course organization, skill laboratory management, course evaluation, extra medical education qualification, medical education research and others. The recognition of such roles will help the appropriate development of all these required activities, which may otherwise be neglected as extra-burden.

5. Individual's mistake, system's error, health safety and trainees

There is still an unacceptably high level of risk associated with medicine, surgery and hospital stays.[59] Medicine remains a high-risk activity because it has not yet assimilated the necessary values to maintain safety practices.[10] A mishap in health setting commonly occurs due to various errors like communication, environmental, human, team-work, technical, instrumental, decision-making, cross-checking, and others. Improvement of all such situation to minimize problems will not adequately occur if the law is to hold individual clinicians responsible for 'mistakes'. To err is human; if humans are solely responsible, then errors will be there. Humans are fallible but the institute or the State should not be. Individual's mistake, system's error and medical negligence are separate entities. When individual's mistake causes harm to patients or others, then it becomes system's error. The institute and the State should continuously evolve foolproof cross-checking methods to prevent individual's mistakes and harm to patients and others, i.e. system's errors. Moreover if a trainee who is not adequately trained makes mistake, should the blame be put on the individual for making the mistake or on the institute or the State for posting or allowing the 'not-adequately' trained personnel to provide such service, i.e. for conducting system's errors? Improvement of any situation and team work requires workshops, training and making guidelines and rules by the institute or the State. The onus for safety should be on the institution and/or the State, rather than on the individuals. The institute or the State then can make enquiry which will also be useful for prevention of such mistakes and errors again. For gross, i.e. not expected considering the level of training of the personnel as per the existing local norms, situation and data, or deliberate medical negligence by the clinicians, the medical council is there to look after. With the responsibility, and the fear, the institutes and the State will gear up to follow all the possible safety measures. It took around 15 years for the modern airline industry to move from being a 'high-risk' industry to becoming a 'safety critical' or 'high reliability' culture. The outcome of this is well evidenced - it is now very safe to fly.[10] The responsibility of airline safety lies with the airline industry and the State, not just on individual pilots. There is a need of developing a fundamental shift in values and practices of the medical education that would transform the safety culture.[10]

5.1 Lesson learned

Lesson 20: Health safety is a responsibility of the institute and the State

Delivery of the health care service to the people is the responsibility of the State. Health service and training of medical professionals are interrelated.[14] Training of medical profession is also the responsibility of the State. Similarly safety of the patients in the health care service is the responsibility of the State and Institute and it cannot be left on the individual health workers or trainees. There are two major safety issues in the health care all over the world. One is to provide the expert assessment and planning of the management of sick patients as early as possible by the already trained faculty and the other is preventing unnecessary procedures, investigations and medications. The medical service in the human society should ultimately aim to provice immediate assessment of every new patient admitted in the hospitals by the already trained faculty twenty four hours a day seven days a week. Such assessment and care could be crucial for the survival of many patients. For the safety of the residents as well, the trainees cannot be just exposed to the situation or practice for which they are not adequately trained. The training should be supervised, structured and graded. Coverage by the trained supervisor and faculty is vital. Residents need also to be trained in all the basic safety principles. Health institutes, medical schools and the State are like industry. They have all the resources and experts to plan, implement and evaluate the safety issues. Service, training, and safety are directly or indirectly dependent on the finance. If optimum service, training, and safety are the responsibility of the institute or the State, not of the individual clinicians, the economic benefits or loss will also relate to the institute or the

State, not to the individual clinicians. If compensations are to be given by the institute or the State, not by the individual practitioners, the benefits, if any!, should also go to the institute or the State. The payment to the individual clinicians will then be as per the service hours, expenses required to acquire the skills and the training, and other factors, not payment according to every procedure. Because outcome of every procedure is also dependent on the patient-selection, quality of the instruments, facilities available, support human resources, team works and other factors, not just on the skill of operator. As such the skill may be difficult to acquire initially. But once acquired, it will be just maintained or improved like driving skill. On the other hand it is not easy to maintain 'knowledge' in this era of information bombardment. The institute or the State has also the responsibility to upgrade the skill and knowledge of the medical practitioners for the sake of the safety of the patients. The medical professionals decide the indication of any procedures and situations should not be created to make them bias in any form. If the operators, surgeons or interventionists are paid for each procedure, there will naturally be the increased probability of advising unnecessary surgeries and procedures not only to the individual patients but also even in the institutional or national guidelines. If the medical professionals who perform the procedures are paid inappropriately high as stipend by the institute, even if not directly for each procedure, it can lead to the similar situation. If the cost and benefit of the procedures is to be borne by the institute, the medical professional can decide the indication without any bias. It is, thus, a very important issue of safety, i.e. rights, of the patients. At this point it would be relevant to emphasize that all the medical professionals themselves also belong to the patient groups, especially in the old age, with consequent liability to the society and the State. The related aspect for the trainee is that if the teachers are paid for the procedure and are biased to perform the procedure, the learning will be similarly acquired, directly or indirectly. The residents ultimately learn considering the actual practice, not just the theoretical teaching or 'preaching', of their teachers. The medical students may from beginning be bias even to choose their career considering the economic benefit, rather than aptitude. Such tendency is observed both in developing and the industrialized countries. In this era of rapid and massive growth of diagnostic and therapeutic technology, unnecessary procedures, investigations, and medications are the major risks to patients as well as the significant cause of economic burden to the insurance companies, the State and ultimately to the people.

6. Conclusion

Medical education has evolved from different models and different educational strategies have been developed considering the experience and evidences. There is continuum of medical education from undergraduate medical education to structured-residential programme of specialist training incorporating the various learning theories. The concept of the structured training programme of residency with actual working in the field under supervision with various teaching-learning and communication activities is to make the learners learn actively and reflectively and be able to perform their responsbilities reflexly professionally. After graduation, all medical professionals need to undergo supervised, structured residential training of actual working and get accredited in the General Specialty like General Surgery, Internal Medicine, General Practice or others. Then only they can either practice in the General Specialty or go for Sub-Specialist Training similarly in different sub-specialties like cardiology, infectious diseases, urology and others. Training in different specialties has to match the community service. The aim of the residential training is to make the medical practitioners fit to practice as per the community need. Public health institutes fulfilling the requirements have to be involved in the residential training programmes. Structured residential training, as well as later revalidation and appraisal, programmes are the responsibilities of the State, not of individual medical institutes or trainees. Committee or councils are required to accredit institutes, like medical schools and public and private institutes, for training and to accredit the structured residential programme.

The educational impact of the assessment on the learning of students is significant and faculty must utilize it to the maximum. Training should be planned focusing on the criterion-referenced assessment. The assessment criteria, especially the eligibility criteria for the exit examination, should be clearly spelled out as per the outcomes we want of the products of the training. Inclusion of training and assessment in communication in the training programme matches the importance of history taking and communication in the actual practice. Establishment of skill lab in developing countries is an urgent responsibility to be fulfilled by the national and international agencies. Considering the vast areas of training requirements in the short period available, the patients' safety, need of training of all the medical graduates in the community and the dearth of the faculty to fulfill the criteria to guide the thesis work, the practice of keeping thesis study of the patients, attending the health institutes primarily for the treatment, in the clinical training programme of the residents is not appropriate. Appropriate training and education of medical professionals are very vital for the safety and care of the patients and the community. Eduction role of medical professionals should be given due priority. Teachers' criteria and training need to match the expected training of the residents and provide the opportunities for training for all the medical graduates in the community. Then only we can expect the practice of EBM from the medical practitioners in every encounter with patients. To achieve such practice of EBM in each and every encounter with patients and to move the medical world from being a high-risk service to becoming a high reliability culture, there appears a fundamental need to acknowledge that health service, medical education and patient safety, and thus the health economics, are all interrelated and are the responsibility of the State, not the individuals.

7. References

[1] Mayer D. Essential Evidence-Based Medicine. 2nd Ed. Cambridge: Cambridge University Press, 2010.

[2] Harden RM, Grant J, Buckley G, Hart IR. Best Evidence Medical Education Guide No. 1. Dundee: Association for Medical Education in Europe, 1999.

[3] Hammick M. Interprofessional education: evidence from the past to guide the future. Medical Teacher 2000;22(5): 461

[4] Harden RM. O:1 Issues in Medical Education: Best Evidence Medical Education. Dundee: Centre for Medical Education, 2005.

[5] Hart IR, Harden RM. Best evidence medical education: a plan for action. Medical Teacher 2000;22(2):131.

[6] Papa FJ, Harasym PH. Medical curriculum reform in North America, 1765 to the present: A cognitive science perspective. Academic Medicine 1999; 74: 154-164.

[7] Harden RM, Sowden S, Dunn WR. Some educationl strategies in curriculum development: The SPICES model. Medical Education, 1984; 18:284-297.

[8] Harden RM, Davis MH, Crosby JR. The new Dundee medical curriculum: a whole that is greater than the sum of the parts. Medical Education 1997;31:264-271,
[9] Law SAT. TL:17 Personal Development Planning. Dundee: Centre for Medical Education, 2008.
[10] Bleakley A, Bligh J, Browne J. Medical Education for the Future: Identity, Power and Location. London: Springer, 2011.
[11] Kaufman DM, Mann KV, Jennet PA. Teaching and Learning in Medical Education: How Theory can Inform Practice. Edinburgh: Association for the Study of Medical Education (ASME); 2000.
[12] Hamdorf JM, Hall C. Acquiring surgical skills. BJS 2000;87:28-37.
[13] McLeod PJ, Harden RM. Clinical Teaching Strategies for Physicians. Medical Teacher 1985;7: 173-89.
[14] Harden RM. Ten questions to ask when planning a course or curriculum. Medical Education 1986;20:356-365.
[15] World Federation for Medical Education. Postgraduate Medical Education: WFME Global Standards for Quality Improvement. Copenhagen: World Federation for Medical Education, 2003.
[16] Accreditation Council for Graduate Medical Education. Bylaws. Illinois: Accreditation Council for Graduate Medical Education, 2011.
[17] Liaison Committee on Medical Education. Rules of Procedure. Washington: Liaison Committee on Medical Education, 2010.
[18] 4 UK Health Departments. Modernising Medical Careers - The Next Steps: The Future Shape of Foundation, Specialist and General Practice Training Programmes. London: Department of Health, 2004.
[19] Harden RM, Crosby JR, Davis MH, Howie PW, Struthers AD. Tasked-based learning: the answer to integration and problem-based learning in the clinical years. Medical Education. 2000; 34: 391-7.
[20] Nepal Medical Council. Regulations for Postgraduate Medical Education (MD/MS Programs). Kathmandu: Nepal Medical Council, 2006.
[21] WHO. World health report 2002: Reducing risks, promoting healthy life. Geneva: WHO, 2003.
[22] Medical Council of India. Postgraduate Medical Education Regulations. New Delhi: Medical Councils of India, 2000.
[23] College of Physicians and Surgeons Pakistan. Guidelines for Examiners. Karachi: College of Physicians and Surgeons Pakistan, 2003.
[24] National Academy of Medical Sciences. Curriculum for MD/MS (as per the specialty). Kathmandu: National Academy of Medical Sciences, 2008.
[25] National Academy of Medical Sciences. Curriculum for DM/MCh (as per the specialty). Kathmandu: National Academy of Medical Sciences, 2011.
[26] Patil NG. The postgraduate curriculum. In: Dent JA, Harden RM, eds. A Practical Guide for Medical Teachers. 2nd Ed. Edinburgh: Elsevier/Churchill Livingstone, 2005: 28-37
[27] Bhattarai MD. Dentistry - a medical specialization. British Dental Journal 2003; 194: 466.
[28] Harden RM. Assess students: An overview. Medical Teacher 1979;1(2): 65-70.
[29] Turnbull JM. What is … normative versus criterion-referenced assessment? Medical Teacher 1989; 11(2): 145-50.
[30] Glasser R. Instructional technology and the measurement of learning outcomes. Am Psychologists. 1963; 18: 519-21.
[31] Steward A. CD:13 Quality Assurance in Medical Education. Dundee: Centre for Medical Education; 2005.

[32] Bhattarai MD. Ten criteria for criterion-referenced assessment in postgraduate MD/MS education. In: Dixit H, Joshi SK. Eds. Modern Trends in Medical Education. Kathmandu: Kathmandu Medical College, 2009: 144-158.
[33] Knowles MS. The Modern Practice of Adult Education: From Pedagogy to Andragogy. New York: Cambridge Books; 1980.
[34] Laidlaw JM, Harden RM. What is ......a study guide? Medical Teacher, 1990;12:7.
[35] Ananthanarayanan PH. Problem based learning. In: Ananthanarayanan N, Sethuraman KR, Kumar S, eds. Pondicherry: Alumni Association of National Teacher Training Centre, JIPMER; 2000. 89-98.
[36] Spencer FC. Teaching and measuring surgical techniques - the technical evaluation of competence. Bulletin of the American College of Surgeons 1978;63:9-12.
[37] Bhattarai MD. General surgery units, asymptomatic gallstones and benign prostatic hypertrophy. The Surgeon - Journal of the Royal College of Surgeons and Edinburgh and Ireland. 2003; 1: 361.
[38] Ziv A. Simulators and simulation-based medical education. In: Dent JA, Harden RM, Eds. A Practical Guide to Medical Teachers. Edinburgh: Churchill Livingstone, 2009: 217-222.
[39] Aly EH. S: 4 Teaching Practical Skills. Dundee: Centre for Medical Education, 2009.
[40] Yaegashi N, Kuramoto M, Nakayama C, Nakano M, Yajma A. Resident gynecologists and total hysterectomy. Tohokti J Exp Med 1996;178:299-306.
[41] Meehan JJ, Georgeson KE. The learning curve associated with laparoscopic antireflux surgery in infants and children. J Pediatric Surgery 1997;32:426-429
[42] Watson DI, Baigrie RJ, Jamieson GG. A learning curve for laparoscopic fundoplication: Definable, avoidable, or a waste of tune? Ann Surg 1996;224:198-203.
[43] Peterson MC, Holbrook JH, Von Hales D, et al. Contributions of the history, physical examination, and laboratory investigation in making medical diagnoses. West J Med 1992;156:163-165.
[44] Reilly BM. Physical examination in the care of medical inpatients: an observational study. Lancet 2003;362:1100-1105.
[45] Cushing A, Mallinson C. Communication. In: Kumar P, Clark M, Eds. 7th Edition. Kumar & Clark's Clinical Medicine. Edinburgh: Saunders Elsevier, 2009: 8-17.
[46] Bhattarai MD. Multiple Choice Questions and Open Ended Questions for Written Assessment. Kathmandu: DMDB 2005.
[47] McAleer S. Choosing assessment instruments. In: Dent JA, Harden RM, eds. A Practical Guide for Medical Teachers. 2nd Ed. Edinburgh: Elsevier/Churchill Livingstone, 2005: 302-310.
[48] Bhattarai MD. Portfolio: Focused on Communication. Kathmandu: National Academy of Medical Sciences, 2007.
[49] Law S, Davis M. TL:13 Portfolio Building. Dundee: Centre of Medical Education 2005.
[50] Neades BL. Professional portfolios: all you need to know and were afraid to ask. Accident and Emergency Nursing 2003; 11: 49-55.
[51] Challis M. AMEE Medical Education Guide No.11 (revised): Portfolio-based learning and assessment in medical education. Medical Teacher 1999; 21(4): 370-85.
[52] Harden RM, Crosby JR. Education Guide No. 20 - The Good Teacher is More Than a Lecturer: The Twelve Roles of the Teacher. Dundee: Association for Medical Education in Europe, 2000.
[53] Bhattarai MD. Study skills course in medical education for postgraduate residents. Kathmandu University Medical Journal 2007; 5(4):561-565.
[54] Bhattarai MD. ABCDEF IS - The principle of constructive feedback. J Nep Med Assoc 2007;46 (167):151-156

[55] Dent J. Education Guide No. 26 : Clinical Teaching in Ambulatory Care Settings - Making the Most of Learning Opportunities with Outpatients. Dundee: Association for Medical Education in Europe, 2006.

[56] Bhattarai MD. Portfolio: Focused on Postgraduate Training. Kathmandu: National Academy of Medical Sciences, 2007.

[57] Royal College of General Practitioners. Quality and Audit in General Practice: Meanings and Definitions. London: Royal College of General Practitioners; 1993.

[58] Bhattarai MD. Ten PM note of organophosphate poisoning: Successful outcome of a medical audit with complete seven steps. J Nep Med Assoc 2010;49(177):76-83.

[59] Amalberti R, Auroy Y. Five system barriers to achieving ultra safe health care. Annals of Internal Medicine, 2005;142:756-764.

4

A Post-Structuralist View of Evidence-Based Medicine (EBM)

Brian Walsh
University of Otago
New Zealand

1. Introduction

Evidence-based medicine has been *praised* for its enormous contribution to information processing, and for other achievements. Most of the *criticism* has been directed at its conceptual structure. This criticism has been levelled by philosophers and doctors, such as Miles, Loughlin and Polychronis. My own approach is to develop a viewpoint on EBM from post-structuralism. I have drawn on the work of Foucault, Deleuze and Guattari, *a celebration of smooth space and nomadic science.* In this chapter I place the doctor with the patient and her problems in smooth space, detour into the striated space of the medical (EBM) gaze, then back into the smooth space of the patient and her problems. I explain "smooth space", "striated space" along with the related concepts of "nomadic science" and "State science", and I explain the "medical gaze" which I update to the "EBM gaze."

1.1 Striated space and smooth space

Deleuze and Guattari provide an account of their division of the universe into the smooth space of the nomad, the war machine and nomadic science, and the striated space instituted by the State apparatus. What might appear a straightforward division quickly reveals a number of complexities. Smooth space and striated space are mixed together and have a moving borderline. The desert becomes mapped, and a city in a declining empire drifts into desert. This transfer from smooth to striated space is a different movement from the transfer from striated to smooth space. By now we can picture a de jure distinction between smooth and striated spaces, and a de facto distinction. The former is abstract. In characterising the two kinds of space, Deleuze and Guattari explain that we occupy smooth space without counting. By contrast, we count in order to occupy striated space. Thus we structure the city before living in it. *Taking the distiction to the level of thought and knowledge,* an example might be the medical thinking of a previous decade in which certain divisions that seemed exclusive and fixed are now blurred - living versus non-living - where do you put prions, parasite versus inclusion - where should we put the viruses that have incorporated themselves into human DNA through the eons of human evolution?

Deleuze and Guattari explain that nomadic science, the science of smooth space, often contributes to major science, renewing it. Even so, minor science would be insipid without the rigour of major or State science. The striation of smooth space is a complex issue. It cannot be done very well: try striating infinity, or the slightest angle of declination. This means that striation is done by verticals and tangents: these cannot gain control of a very small angle. Nor can lamination, the process used in striation, control smooth space at a macroscopic level. At the other pole, it escapes them by the spiral or vortex, in other words, a figure in which all the points of space are simultaneously occupied according to the laws of frequency or of accumulation, distribution; these laws are distinct from the so-called laminar distribution corresponding to the striation of parallels.[1] Using a mathematical model, they tell us that the striation of smooth space EBM, which I depict as an aspect of State science, tries to striate the smooth space of medical practice, and I argue that this can be done only incompletely.

> *...is an operation that undoubtedly consists in subjugating, overcoding, metricising smooth space, in neutralising it, but also in giving it a milieu of propagation, extension, refraction, renewal, and impulse without which it would perhaps die of its own accord:...".*[2]

1.2 State science and nomadic science

Deleuze and Guattari explain that, from the point of view of the State apparatus, the war machine appears in negative form: "stupidity, deformity, madness, illegitimacy, usurpation, sin." The war machine betrays everything. Deleuze and Guattari go on to explain the *difficulty in conceiving of the war machine*. It is everywhere exteriority - the unfamiliar and wild or unstructured - , whereas the State apparatus is everywhere interiority, what we are accustomed to, and from which we take our point of view. They depict the war machine in terms of the expression of feeling which then becomes affect. Projected with velocity, this affect of love or hate becomes exterior.

Deleuze and Guattari introduce epistemology here. There is, they tell us, a scientific dimension to the conflict between 1) the State/interiority and 2) the war machine/exteriority. Deleuze and Guattari[3] distinguish a State science from nomadic science, or minor science, or at least a way of treating science. The former is the traditional science, hallowed by the State, but the latter is not supported by history, law, or royal authority. Because nomadic science does not develop from a recognized centre, Deleuze and Guattari refer to it as "eccentric science", and set out four characteristics. It posits a fluid model rather than a solid/fluid model--"Flux is reality itself".[4] Secondly, the eccentric scientific model depicts becoming and heterogeneity, rather than fixed scientifically investigable types with their "homogeneity" within categories for the purpose of grouping and generalizing. This contrasts with the stability and constancy in the State science model. Thirdly, rather than occupying a rectangular, striated space, the eccentric science involves a vortical (like a vortex) movement in open space. There are flows in smooth space. This contrasts with State science in striated space, which is set out in matrix form before use. Fourthly, the eccentric science is occupied with problems produced by affect – the restless desire to be able to do certain things. Working towards their solutions is the task of the war machine. The pathway is punctuated by accidents, movements, change, and is typified by events, rather than essences. The nomad signifier is essentially disruptive, and is like a tent—temporary, shifting, adjusting to local conditions, but providing a kind of shelter within

[1] Deleuze and Guattari 1987, p. 489.

[2] Deleuze and Guattari 1987, p. 486.

[3] 1987, pp. 361 ff.

[4] Deleuze and Guattari 1987, p. 361.

which state-like processes can go on. By contrast, the State science is immersed in rationality - like a house or castle or farm with fences.

The war machine is projected into an abstract knowledge which is developing away from the centre of the State science, and which is formalised differently from the State science. (For example, this eccentric science relates differently to technology.) The State science has a complex relationship with the nomad or minor science.[5] The State science partly excludes and belittles the minor science, (describing it as a "prescientific, parascientific or subscientific agency"[6]) but otherwise dominates it, siphoning off some of its results and its thinkers. These latter are then in a state of imbalance between being 1) energised by the war machine and 2) saturated with rationality. The minor science pressurises the State science, which sometimes yields, to a degree, incorporating some of the viewpoint of the minor science, structuring this new material in its own fashion. Symmetrically, the minor science detaches aspects of the State science. The upshot of these gains and losses is that the border is always changing, as is the uneasy relationship between EBM, academic medicine, dissenters from the dominant paradigm, and real practice.

One of the discordant differences between State science and minor science lies in the division of labour, which is largely determined by the pattern of scientific activity. State science and minor science divide their labour differently. For example, there are differences in the type and level of skill, and in the numbers of workers, and their geographic distribution. This is one of the reasons why State science resists minor science. Any gain in ground made by minor science involves a change in the distribution of labour. This can have profound economic and social implications, and is likely to be resisted with all the might of capitalism. An example would be the promotion of meditation as a substitute for tranquillizers.

State science has been developed around gravity, seriousness and rectitude. This is related to the arborescent form of knowledge and the structuring logos of rectitude. This vertical force has led the way to the concepts of "parallel" and "horizontal". These are derived from the vertical force of gravity.

> *Homogeneous space is in no way a smooth space; on the contrary, it is the form of striated space. The space of pillars. It is striated by the fall of bodies, the verticals of gravity, the distribution of matter into parallel layers, the lamellar and laminar movement of flows.*[7]

Over the centuries scientists and mathematicians have developed a striated space, bringing in Euclidian geometry. They have identified the straight line as the shortest path between

---

[5] Nomadic science is science which cannot firmly plant its roots in any particular well structured scientific discourse because the ontology or metaphysics of those discourses do not adequately capture the things, explanations and phenomena that one needs to be able to understand. Nomadic science therefore takes resources where it can and uses them in ways that the contributing disciplines would find undisciplined because it asks poorly formed questions that do not properly respect the current contours of debate. For instance, when one asks how the legislative context and the political emancipation of women affects the biology of the HIV virus this sounds like an illegitimate question. Or if one asks how the MAO levels available in the amygdala of the right temporal lobe are influenced by a history of colonization, that sounds equally flaky and disruptive or destructive in terms of orderly, striated science ("Personal Communication", Gillett, 2010).

[6] Deleuze and Guattari 1987, p. 367.

[7] Deleuze and Guattari 1987, p. 370.

two points, and the "multiplicities termed metric or arborescent".[8] By now we have a space which is homogeneous, and visual. Of great importance is the universal attraction between two bodies. With these principles, any part of the world can be a striated space, the striation not being tied to any one part of the earth. Whenever a new field of science arises, royal science tries to mould the new science into this homogeneous structure. Deleuze and Guattari state that chemistry moved forward once the concept of weight had been elaborated.[9]

Nomadic science is not like this. While it does not refute gravity and its associated phenomena, it is not dependent on them, and cannot be reduced to them. It lodges in a supplement or excess, over and above gravity and is correlates. A fundamental departure was the slightest excess of angle, the slightest deviation from the straight line. Take, for example, a body which falls along a curved path. *This freedom allows nomadic science to reach into unstructured areas.* By now we have the space of the smallest deviation, and this is smooth space.

> *...therefore it has no homogeneity, except between infinite proximate points, and the linking of proximities is effected independently of any determined path. It is a space of contact, of small tactile or manual actions of contact, rather than a visual space like Euclid's striated space.*[10]

Smooth space is heterogeneous and occupied by different multiplicities. These are acentred and rhizomatic. Deleuze and Guattari apply the words *rapidity* and *celerity*[11] to movement which deviates even minimally. As pointed earlier, this movement is vortical (as in a vortex or spiral) and actually draws smooth space. "All the points of space are simultaneously occupied according to the laws of frequency or of accumulation, distribution; these laws are distinct from the so-called laminar distribution corresponding to the striation of parallels".[12] EBM, so structured, cannot reach into all of smooth space, and so cannot relate adequately to the partly disorganized world of human health, with its polyglot forces. In fact, the qualitative opposition gravity-celerity, slow-rapid, heavy-light is coextensive with science but does not constitute a quantitative part of it. Rather it provides a space for distinguishing between striated space and smooth space, and it regulates their interaction, including the domination of one by the other.

Royal science is characterised by reproduction, while nomad science allows thought to get away from the traditional base, such as *the subject*, or *humanity*, and to wander freely, to create new areas.[13] In royal science, then, there is enough lattice-work to provide for constant relations between variables and continuity between competing representations. Deduction and induction are possible. For reproduction to occur, a fixed point of reference is available from which to view the process. These are not the processes of itinerant or

---

[8] Deleuze and Guattari 1987, p. 370.

[9] 1987, p. 370.

[10] The use of a straight line to limn a curve is well characterized mathematically by means of tangents, as Aristotle notes, but the use of a curve to map another curve is not well established and so with smooth or nomadic science there may not be striated or well organized relationships of mapping between the discourse and its structures of meaning and the phenomenon of interest.

[11] Swiftness.

[12] Deleuze and Guattari 1987, p. 489.

[13] Colebrook 2002, p. xxvii.

nomadic science, which moves in smooth space, in search of singularities of matter or material, rather than form. The meaning of the world changes. This is because the deterritorialization creates the territory. Instead of calculating constants which bind variables, nomad science tracks the variations of the variables, as in language.

The State science is always trying to striate the smooth space. A multiplicity in smooth space is at risk of having a grid of parallel vectors superimposed. Then it can be visualised from a vantage point. By contrast, nomadic science would have followed the multiplicity "in an 'exploration by legwork'".[14] The nomad science tries to retain or regain its smooth space, where it can follow the singularities in vortical flows. State science is often interacting in complex ways with the leaders of nomadic science, sometimes conferring a minor position in its system upon one of them.

State science, including experimental science, have considerable conceptual equipment and metric power, but ambulant sciences are not able to evolve autonomy. Always in problematic mode, they draw, and link up, smooth space. They follow the flow of matter, and so stay with reality. However, the modus operandi of State science is to extract operations from intuition, setting up categorised structures. Some resources are devoted to safety, as in the building of a bridge from diagrams. By contrast, nomadic science's problem-solving modus operandi often takes it into uncharted territory as it moves from singularity to singularity. With regard to the inattention to safety as nomadic science proceeds, it is likely to have to sort out the consequences in real life. Deleuze and Guattari[15] explain that nomadic science works, often intuitively, among problems, but often needs the resources of State science to structure and solve these.

Underlying these considerations is the layer of reality called "thought". Bear in mind that Deleuze and Guattari consider thought to be an active ingredient of life. (So it would be more accurate to place thought "within these considerations".) These authors depict a circular relationship between the State and thought. All thought conforms to a model of thought produced by the State. But surely we have a way of thinking about the State? But we are told how to do that. So which comes first?[16] They proceed to describe two heads of thought. "There is an imperium of true thinking.....constituting the efficacy of a foundation (mythos); a republic of free spirits proceeding by pact or contract...(logos)".[17] For example, an organism has a lawlike operation that can be studied within its own boundaries as a homeostatic system. (This is related to the episteme of ideal rationality which neglects the relationship between power and knowledge.)

Deleuze and Guattari go on to explain the benefits of this symbiosis. From the State, thought gains gravity. Actually, its heaviness takes thought out of the daily arena, to some extent. Then it goes unchallenged, and with it the benefits to the State. Perhaps it goes unnoticed that the State-form has a consensus. How, without thought, could we fabricate a notion of a State possessed of "de jure universality".[18] So the State alone divides subjects into "rebel" and "supportive". Taking advantage of the status of reason, the State characterises itself as

[14] Deleuze and Guattari 1987, p. 373.
[15] 1987, p. 374.
[16] Deleuze and Guattari 1987, p. 374.
[17] Deleuze and Guattari 1987, p. 375.
[18] p. 375.

"the rational and reasonable organization of the community".[19] Drawing on the power of the State, reason is fleshed out as the State. "It was all over the moment the State-form inspired an image of thought. With full reciprocity".[20]

Deleuze and Guattari[21] amalgamate exterior thought and the war machine, in their model. Describing noology as the study of thought images, they explain that "outside thought can disturb the results of this endeavour. They explain that relating these nomadic, scattered thoughts to forces, is not straightforward. For example, Nietzsche's aphorisms, as distinct from maxims, await being operationalized by forces (people). The are calculatedly disruptive and challenging.

> *You shall be such for me that your eye is always seeking an enemy—your enemy. And with some of you there is hate at first sight.*
> *You shall seek your enemy, you shall wage your war—and for your own thoughts!*[22]

Certain forces (people) will convert these thoughts into a war machine. Thus Deleuze and Guattari introduce a diachronic dimension to the amalgamation of nomadic thought into a war machine. Occupying smooth space, these outside thoughts do not function in a method, as in striated space. The arrow (thought) does not move from point to point. It is taken up at any point to be sent to any other point. The points are determined by the change in direction of the thought, or the creation of one thought from another, not vice versa. The thoughts are primary, the points secondary. This resembles the movement of nomads.

States must gain control of smooth space, if possible. For example, they set up systems to control the movement of ships on the sea, especially the Suez canal, because that is a vital junction that controls movement among major domains of opportunity and they police the airways. During the cold war, it was unacceptable for a Russian fighter plane to fly through the air above the USA. As part of this process of extending its communication channels safely through smooth space, the State acts against nomadic movements. This is all part of their aim to control all flows, everywhere. Those movements which are allowed are assessed on several parameters, such as proximity to striated space, speed and direction. These are relativized to the striated space. Here Deleuze and Guattari write of deterritorialization of the earth: when States acquire control over smooth space, they pay little attention to the details of the subordinated nomads, who may themselves be attuned to the reality of the smooth space. An example would be the use of intravenous Vitamin C in the critical zone of the Intensive Care Unit (ICU).[23]

In section one I have given a post-structuralist account of smooth space/striated space and of nomadic science/State science. I have taken the view that EBM is an aspect of State science which provides no account of nomadic science or smooth space. As far as possible these should be supplanted. I place the doctor and patient with her problems in this smooth space, starting this chapter. I now proceed to the medical gaze/EBM gaze which I depict as striated and striating.

---

[19] p. 375.
[20] An example of this reciprocity would be between funding and the biomedical model such that more wild and singular explorations are marginalised.
[21] 1987, pp. 376-7.
[22] Nietzsche 2005, p 41.
[23] Gillett 2011, p. 8.

2. The medical gaze

2.1 The configuration of disease: The space of pathology

Once pathological anatomy had attained high status in the nineteenth century, the space of configuration of disease became superimposed on the body (where it remains). The medical gaze superimposes pathology on anatomy: for instance, a histopathologist looks down a microscope and "recognises" a tubercle, a lesion pathognomonic for tuberculosis. With her training in pathology, she extrapolates from the tubercle under the lens to the disease configuration called "tuberculosis". Foucault says of the sovereign moment of diagnosis,

> *The "glance" has simply to exercise its right of origin over truth.*
> *But how did this supposedly natural, immemorial right come about? How was this locus, in which disease indicated its presence, able to determine in so sovereign a way the figure that groups its elements together?*[24]

The space of the configuration of disease has several principles. The knowledge is historical. This means that over, say, two days, a range of symptoms and signs manifests itself to the clinical gaze. Secondly, the *cause* is in the same space as *effect* but Foucault depicts this space without a temporal dimension so that time does not figure in this model. In this model of the configuration of the disease, "There is only one plane and one moment".[25] (Bear in mind that "disease" is an abstraction, like a map. "Disease" is a conceptual system, a reification of a dynamic process which may or may not share some core features, across individuals--one that we happen to be good at picking up.) A third principle is: "It is a space in which analogies define essences".[26] This means that the differences between two diseases, such as pneumonia and influenza, is established by analogy through the extent to which their surface pictures resemble each other (both exhibit fever and cough, but sputum or the presence of basal crepitations[27] characterise only pneumonia). Lastly, Foucault explains how patient and doctor are interlopers in the disease process or space. Each specific patient distorts the ideal picture of the disease because the patient both reveals and conceals the disease, and the doctor is in a strange situation using her knowledge of disease as a guide, in that she never experiences the disease in ideal form. The doctor chases the disease through her patient who distorts the ideal form. In order to know the truth of the pathological fact the doctor must abstract the patient.[28] What is more, as soon as the doctor begins treatment, she further distorts the disease, if the treatment is effective.

If Foucault is correct, then it is very difficult to practise "patient-centered care" (PCC), which has been defined as "quality healthcare achieved through a partnership between informed and respected patients and their families, and a co-ordinated healthcare team".[29] The practice of PCC is difficult because of the nature and complexity of the diagnostic process. Using her knowledge of pathology as a map or guide, the doctor goes on a hunt for one or another disease or map defined in relation to others by comparison and contrast. But, as

---

[24] 1994, p. 4.
[25] 1994, p. 6.
[26] 1994, p. 6.
[27] These are fine crackles heard, often at the lowest part of a lung.
[28] Foucault 1994, p. 8.
[29] In a 2004 study of patient-centred care, the American National Health Council defined PCC (alfutures.com).

explained in the previous paragraph, the patient a) obscures and b) distorts the ideal picture the doctor is trying to bring into bold relief, although the patient also, perhaps reluctantly, reveals the disease. Using shingles (Herpes Zoster) as an example, the patient may obscure the disease by presenting with pain in the renal area. Many doctors make the wrong diagnosis before the characteristic rash arrives on about the fourth day. With regard to the distortion each patient makes, a doctor may be accustomed to seeing shingles in elderly patients. But if the patient with a painful rash is ten 10 years old, the diagnosis is difficult. (Of course, if the correct diagnosis is made, then the patient has revealed the disease.) Continuing with my assertion that the diagnostic process makes it hard to practise patient-centered care, Foucault explains that the doctor is constantly seeking lacunae. She thinks in the space between true and false (for example, hyperventilation due to anxiety *or* metabolic acidosis), and in the space between viral and bacterial, and in the space between benign and malignant, and in other spaces. This difficult thinking, which surely distracts from thinking about the patient only or the patient at the centre of the process, can be pictured in a space between obscurity and clarity of the disease. In this space is the interaction between the body and the disease. It does not fit the ideal forms captured in the canonical texts and treated with canonical methods. Thus I have postulated a tension between the primary space of pathology and the secondary space of the individual person, as set out by Foucault in *The Birth of the Clinic.*

2.2 The medical gaze in more detail

2.2.1 History

Canguilhem[30] and Foucault extensively develop the space of perception. The term used here is "gaze". The gaze is the perception of the doctor, perceiving the patient, and is scopic or visual. This is because, since the end of the eighteenth century, the post-mortem examination--which is visual--has fundamentally determined how doctors view the diseased patient. Doctors look back from death, in which medical truth is revealed, to life. Secondarily, Foucault allows both auditory and tactile modes of perception to intertwine with vision in the gaze so that a doctor examining a patient's chest might look at the breathing rate, touch the pulsation of the lowermost, leftmost point of distinct cardiac pulsation, and listen to the breath sounds, the three forms of perception functioning together. However, the sight--hearing--touch perception system is subject to the absolute gaze of knowledge. This latter is dominated by death, in that, as previously explained, the post-mortem examination is the foundation stone of medical epistemology.

2.2.2 Pathology dominates the gaze. A new role for death. Medical epistemology modernised

Foucault makes three very interesting points about this imperious, death-infiltrated, gaze. The first is that "The 'glance' has become a complex organization with a view to a spatial assignation of the invisible".[31] "The structure, at once perceptual and epistemological, that commands clinical anatomy, and all medicine that derives from it, is that of *invisible visibility*".[32] A doctor (and this is the second point) is drawing a 3D picture, not learning,

[30] 1978.

[31] Foucault 1994, p. 164.

[32] Foucault 1994, p. 165.

when she steadies her gaze on the patient. Obviously, the doctor detects from the 2D surface (usually: sometimes the doctor conducts an internal examination, for example of the rectum, after which she is no longer limited to a 2D assessment) of the body a few clues, through sight, hearing and touch. (When a doctor hears a certain type of murmur between the first and second heart sounds, she may visualise a narrowed space between the cusps of the mitral valve. When she palpates the lowermost, leftmost point of distinct cardiac pulsation and finds it is further to the left than normal, she visualises an enlarged heart.) The gaze uses knowledge of human life, derived from post-mortem examination, to build a 3D (functional) model of the body's disease. This aspect of the Foucaldian gaze is important with regard to EBM because its epistemology assumes that the 3D picture is objective. But it implicitly undermines EBM evidence in that EBM evidence provides *a* truth, rather than *the* truth. After all, each doctor might build a different 3D model. A third interesting point made by Foucault about the gaze is that it medicalises the human world. This means that people are now viewed in a dichotomy of diseased--healthy whereby "....one did not think first of the internal structure of *the organized being*, but of the *medical bipolarity of the normal and the pathological*".[33] EBM has inherited this powerful bias, this binary thinking, not that of life and health and normal living.

I have indicated that the post-mortem examination laid the foundation of the medical gaze which henceforth would establish disease as individual and require a nuanced use of the old language to express the newly perceived realities of pathological anatomy in combination with the age-old symptoms. However, Foucault explains two other developments arising from the use of the post-mortem examination. One is that death, as well as being individualised, was also concretised. It moved into the space previously occupied by the gods and immortality. There was a decrease in theory and systems that had befuddled earlier generations of doctors.

Early in the nineteenth century in France, the belief that disease had an essence which "was both nature and counter-nature",[34] was removed from the medical gaze. To constitute the new gaze then, the post-mortem examination had to form or inform the foundation of medical epistemology--

> *In anatomical perception, death was the point of view from the height of which disease opened up onto truth; the life/disease/death trinity was articulated in a triangle whose summit culminated in death; perception could grasp life and disease in a single unity only insofar as it invested death in its own gaze.*[35]

From early in the nineteenth century, death built into the gaze a better understanding of life and disease, using the anatomical--clinical model. Death also built into the gaze the dissolution of disease, and the limited nature of disease as that which enabled death, rather than death being the consequence of disease. Thus the medical gaze is henceforth structured to regard death as more fundamental than disease, which death elucidates (through post-mortem examination) and terminates (hence it is basilisk-like).

---

[33] Foucault 1994, p. 35.
[34] Foucault 1994, p. 155.
[35] Foucault 1994, p. 158.

The epistemological foundation stone for this view of disease is, by now, the post-mortem examination and from that origin the gaze proceeds to construct the individual. Previously, clinical medicine had dealt with cases. But the new gaze is to be different. The post-mortem examination provides information about the individual so disease is primarily the disease of an individual. It is no longer the case that each individual presents a variation on a general phenomenon. Thus the idea that the individual is an exemplar of a general phenomenon is now problematised.

2.2.3 The gaze is multifaceted

The gaze is "not content to observe what was self-evident".[36]

Foucault explains that the gaze involves possibilities and probabilities, risks--and experience. He reminds us that society confers authority on the doctor, so that the doctor from her gaze, announces the truth (The doctor says she has cancer: so she has cancer).

> *In the clinic, it was a question of a much more subtle and complex structure in which the integration of experience occurred in a gaze that was at the same time knowledge, a gaze that exists, that was master of its truth .... . . At this level there was no distinction to be made between theory and experience, method and results; one had to read the deep structures of visibility in which field and gaze are bound together by codes of knowledge;...the linguistic structure of the sign and the aleatory structure of the case.*[37]

2.2.4 Disease is now visible, but needs to be articulated

Here Foucault draws attention to the need for a language that relates the signs and symptoms of diseases to human understanding and communication. This matter belongs in linguistic and semiological spaces. Bear in mind that the gaze includes questioning the patient, in language. The patient answers verbally and non-verbally. Foucault explains that language needed to adapt to the new knowledge so that the disease of the individual could be seen. Doctors who conducted the post-mortem examinations needed to clothe the new knowledge in words that would convey it to absent clinicians:-

> *It is no longer a question of correlating a perceptual sector and a semantic element, but of bending language back entirely towards that region in which the perceived, in its singularity, runs the risk of eluding the form of the word and of becoming finally imperceptible because incapable of being said.*[38]

Foucault tells us how the language was adapted to express the new perceptions "to introduce language into that penumbra where the gaze is bereft of words".[39] He mentions the use of colour, metaphor, empirical comparisons, the value of intersensorial qualities, and references to the normal and everyday. Many of these ways of making the perceived expressible were deployed by Laennec, whose early description of one cirrhotic liver, quoted by Foucault, exemplifies these linguistic developments.

---

[36] Foucault 1994, p. 89.
[37] pps. 81, 90.
[38] Foucault 1994, p. 169.
[39] 1994, p. 169.

The liver...when cut, it seemed to be made up entirely of a mass of small seeds, round or oval in shape, varying in size from a millet seed to a hemp seed. These seeds, which can be easily separated, left almost no gap between them in which one might be able to make out some remaining part of the real tissue of the liver; they were fawn or reddish-yellow in colour, verging in parts on the greenish; their fairly moist, opaque tissue was slack, rather than soft, to touch, and when one squeezed the grains between one's fingers only a small part was crushed, the rest feeling like a piece of soft leather.[40]

I have alluded obscurely to an issue which needs clarifying. In Foucault, a distinction is made between a statement and the visible. I have explained that when the post-mortem examinations were first used to provide knowledge, it was necessary to develop a language--statements--to match the visible. Foucault provides an account of the difference in the nature of these two, the visible and the articulable. Read what Deleuze explains regarding Foucaldian theory:

...there is a difference in nature between the form of content and the form of expression, between the visible and the articulable (although they continually overlap and spill into one another in order to compose each stratum or form of knowledge). ...Between the two there is no isomorphism or conformity, in spite of a mutual presupposition and the primacy of the statement. ...there is neither causality from one to the other nor symbolization between the two, and that if the statement has an object, it is a discursive object which is unique to the statement and is not isomorphic with the visible object. Of course we dream of isomoprhism, ..."[41]

I consider that all this eludes EBM. Does this matter? I argue that EBM rides rapidly over some deep and obscure issues yet urges us to change the way we treat sick people. EBM moves the articulable around from paper to paper and book to book to guidelines, but I suspect that these writers assume that the object of the statement is the visible object: I am sure that EBM protagonists assume that what we are saying matches what we are seeing. In simple terms, then, I am arguing that such complex, underlying issues make the strident assertions of EBM protagonists seem too strident.

2.2.5 Reconfiguration of the doctor, patient, consultation and epistemology

The other consequence of the new perceptual structure was that this visual system rested on an opaque base. This means that what lay beyond the base was not available for the constitution of knowledge. This is of enormous importance for EBM. Foucault postulates that a change in doctor/patient relationship has occurred over recent centuries in which the key element is epistemology. He uses the metaphor of a grid. By now doctor, patient and their interaction take place in this new grid. This is like children moving their game to a jungle gym. However, no analogy is complete, and, in fact, the children are newly configured (their bodies can go through different sequences), as well as playing by different rules which have resulted from a fundamentally different knowledge that the jungle gym prescribes. This is like a discipline that introduces a new habitas, like the posture associated with ballet.

Previously the doctor and patient were taken as given, not as problematic, although this is an exaggeration. Medical progress was considered to have occurred between the two

[40] Laennec, R. 'De l'auscultation mediate', vol. 1, p. 368.

[41] Deleuze 2006, p. 61.

"givens". For example, early in the twentieth century it became possible for a doctor to arrange for the patient's chest to be X-Rayed. But against this given-ness of the doctor and patient, both were constructions in flux. Late-twentieth-century patients began to manage their own asthma and diabetes, and the doctors also changed. Early in the twentieth century a chest physician had skills to map out the tuberculous cavities in the chest, with whispering pectoriloquy, percussion, and auscultation for bronchial breathing. The late-twentieth-century chest physician had lost some of these skills, but become expert in reading a chest X-Ray film. The chest physician had become subject--in turn--to the gaze. This applies with more force to the cardiologist and neurologist with electrocardiograms, ectroencephalograms, ultra-sound, magnetic resonance imaging and computerised axial tomography.

The space between doctor and patient changed to further complexify the shifting relationships. The physician moved closer to the patient, beginning to examine the rectum and vagina, and to pass a sigmoidoscope into the colon. These procedures brought the interior more directly under the scopic gaze.[42] But further even again to these profound changes from a more subtle and profound level, Foucault challenges this "given", unproblematic nature of the doctor, patient, and consultation space. In the last two decades, EBM has further reconstructed the patient, doctor and intervening space reconstructing the smooth and striated yet again:--[43]

> *A more precise historical analysis reveals a quite different principle of adjustment beyond these adjustments: it bears jointly on the type of objects to be known, on the grid that makes it appear, isolates it, and carves up the elements relevant to a possible epistemic knowledge (savoir), on the position that the subject must occupy in order to map them, on the instrumental mediations that enables it to grasp them, on the modalities of registration and memory that it must put into operation, and on the forms of conceptualization that it must practice and that qualify it as a subject of legitimate knowledge. What is modified in giving place to anatomo-clinical medicine is not, therefore, the mere surface contact between the knowing subject and the known object; it is the more general arrangement of knowledge that determines the reciprocal positions and connexion between the one who must know and that which is to be known. The access of the medical gaze into the sick body was not... it was the result of a recasting at the level of epistemic knowledge (savoir) itself, and not at the level of accumulated, refined, deepened, adjusted knowledge (connaissances).*[44]

The EBM clinician makes little use of herself as a person.[45] Although her reality is with her patient, she quickly sets out on a conceptual trajectory which distances her from her patient. She first asks what group of **P**atients or experimental subjects her patient can be placed in. Then her mind continues to function at a distance from her patient by asking what **I**ntervention she should consider. Third, her mind continues at a distance by asking what intervention is probably less suitable, for **C**omparison. Lastly, she projects herself out of the here and now by asking what **O**utcome, in the future, she is planning. This is the scheme for the PICO question, the start of the EBM process.

The modern (EBM) patient is biomedical, hopefully has one acute disease, depictable though the science of pathology, and is viewed against a background of one or more groups of similar patients whose disease has been investigated through one or more RCTs and/or

[42] The physician moved to the other side.
[43] Of course, Foucault is writing of the early nineteenth century in France.
[44] Foucault 1994, p. 137.
[45] I draw on Wifstad 2008 for this line of thinking.

observational studies. Suitable treatment is available, and affordable. The modern (EBM) doctor is steeped in the studies and/or their downstream proliferations. She sees her patient against a background of groups of experimental subjects whose similarity to her patient she is assessing. Where possible, she is applying clinical guidelines. The space between doctor and patient is infiltrated with research/statistics, and the computer/internet. This is how the grid is constructed. Doctor and patient have moved towards the model of experimenter and experimental subject.

All parties work in a grid of knowledge that has been, or should have been, reconceived, not just increased. The legitimated knowledge is computerised biomedicine, connecting a biomedical patient with a guidelined doctor. This legitimated knowledge has been produced by biomedicine's emblematic group, the protagonists of EBM—a group that has determined what counts as knowledge, who speaks authoritatively, and in particular, what counts as evidence, and what does not. Critically important are the reliability of evidence, the strength of the recomendations flowing from the evidence, and the power/knowledge supporting these.

Foucault makes the point that the sciences of Man and the notion of the uniqueness of Man and his individual qualities, separating him from nature and so on, were not so-called ground-breaking "discoveries". The "Enlightenment" did not "roll back the frontiers of ignorance" and provide a means of knowing the "truth". The "truth" was the product of discourse. Discourses may be understood as bodies of knowledge or disciplines, in themselves the form of disciplinary practices.[46] A discourse enables and limits what can be thought, said and written during a period of time. Discourses produce knowledges and knowledge is made known historically. The historical constitution of knowledge undermines any claim that knowledge is impartial or better than previous knowledge. Foucault does not see an extra-discourse point from which we can assess the correctness of any discourse. Thus the truth about "Man" is not a pale reflection of a real, natural man, idealised in form and content but the actual, engaged, situated human beings described in social sciences and works of art.

It is my contention that EBM does not acknowledge the Foucaldian insight that EBM does not investigate and treat an objective patient, through an objective doctor. Foucault would argue that EBM has constructed the patient, the doctor, and the consultation space. As stated above, EBM has not just added to our knowledge, EBM has set up a new knowledge. And not only that. EBM has established itself as the creator of knowledge, has decided how knowledge is legitimated (through RCTs and observational studies leading on to an hierarchy of evidence and the strength of recommendations flowing from the evidence). It is my contention that all this floats free of evidence, and that the medical profession has not debated it to an agreed conclusion.[47] You could say that EBM has not just altered the goalposts. It has moved us to a new football field and reconfigured the teams and the rules. And yet in some ways EBM plays as if we were on the old field (realistically or mind-independently construed). It's proponents do not acknowledge the constructed status of the patient, the doctor and the consultation space. They do not acknowledge that the patient is set up in terms of variables and mechanisms which EBM can investigate and treat. The investigating gaze of the EBM doctor takes itself to be dividing even to the joints and marrow of nature itself ("cutting nature at the joints"), armed with the spirit of truth.

---

[46] Coveney 2006, p. 4.

[47] Miles et al. 2008, p. 621.

With regard to health care research, the topics selected for investigation will need to fall within the area of intersection of the gaze and health care. The EBM doctor will look for problems suitable for investigation (which assumes funding) through RCT or observational study. Typically this will involve holding one or more variables constant while altering one or more other variables. Obviously, this assumes that such variables can be isolated and dealt with. But there are many aspects of health care which would struggle to fit into this model. For example, palliative care has developed a discourse of dying. There is now a right way to die: quietly. Patients should realise that there comes a stage when definitive treatment should yield to symptomatic treatment. Patients should be actively involved in decisions. But some patients reject this modern discourse on dying. I am not sure that EBM investigates ways a team steeped in the palliative care discourse can work together to support this recalcitrant patient. An issue here for EBM is that the team may be divided as to how to proceed.

Gillett[48] gives an account of HIV/AIDS as a postmodern illness which reveals the limitations of biomedicine, and therefore EBM. In the West, at any rate, the illness follows a period in which traditional values were challenged. This means that some men formed sexual relationships with other men. Other people injected drugs intravenously. These choices confronted the power of biology, in that some people developed HIV/AIDS. Despite extensive research, the (biomedical) treatment for this condition is only partly effective. Sufferers were forced together to try to deal with prevention and education and to support each other in grief. This group of people, accustomed to challenging the social hierarchy, developed partnerships with their health providers, negotiating treatment. Doctors and sufferers had to face the question of whether to tell the partner that the patient had tested positive. Ethical questions arose over testing people for the virus. Although I have referred to the West, the condition spread extensively in the third world. In Africa, Gillett[49] tells us, some men enjoyed their sex with or without the preparedness of the woman. Women often have little education, political power, or rights within the marriage. This all facilitated the spread of infection among women, and therefore among men and children. An ethical issue arose over research into this condition. Largely led by Western organisations, any such research in third world countries was bedevilled by the fact that those who took part in the research were unlikely to be able to afford its benefits. In one study, some desperate research subjects managed to decipher the code in the RCT and break protocol by handing around the active moiety. The point I am making is that there is a (disease) space in which culture and biomedicine meet. With Gillett,[50] I submit that much of what I have described is poorly handled by EBM, whose gaze is restricted—EBM is blind to certain aspects of the problem that is human disease and therefore it may be blind to critical determinants that will make a real difference to the suffering caused. Then with Foucault, I draw attention to the dominance of the narrow EBM discourse and to the association of knowledge and power. The western biomedical gaze constructed our solutions in terms of pharmaceutical remedies rather than in terms of socio-political change, revealing the hegemony of the biomedical, pathological anatomy gaze.

---

[48] 2004, Chapter 8.
[49] 2004.
[50] 2004.

The medical gaze has been said to discriminate against some patients. Such issues as social class, gender, race and whether the patient is paying, have received comment. The medical gaze struggles with comorbidity, and with poorly defined problems and language problems. The medical gaze also struggles with the fact that the modern equivalent of the Hippocratic airs and spaces is to widen our gaze to the socio-culturo-politico-historical contexts of disease. As stated above, this last struggle has implications for patients with AIDS, for example.

The gaze surely includes the higher valuation which doctors place on signs as distinct from symptoms. This is described by Foucault,[51]who explains how numerous chest diseases can be heralded by such symptoms as cough and shortness of breath. However, early in the nineteenth century, Laennec focused on examination of the chest. He found that, in a few patients, the voice was transmitted surprisingly well to a small area of the chest wall. He called this clinical sign "pectoriloquy", and made the (epistemological) decision that this, rather than the symptoms, would establish the diagnosis (of Pulmonary Tuberculosis). To this day doctors prioritise signs (and particularly images and the results of laboratory investigations with their attached figures) over symptoms if they point to different diagnoses. In passing I note the very interesting point that Laennec made an epistemological leap. However, the point of this paragraph is simply to flesh in Foucault's medical gaze with more detail.

2.2.6 EBM rhetoric

EBM exaggerates the importance of its "gold standard" evidence in the EBM gaze. During the (PICO) conceptual excursion, the doctor needs look back at her patient and assess the patient's suitability for this research-based intervention. EBM leaders have, in 2008, provided detailed guidance on this. There is a complex issue regarding the judgment as to whether the patient is suitable for the intervention, the alternative, and even the outcome proposed. The doctor must know something of the patient, her attitudes, values, preferences, and perhaps even her social situation. With increasing emphasis on the business aspect of medicine and also the scientific aspect and the computer, this detailed understanding of the patient is declining in comparison to what it was in the time when most people lived in a country district and saw one doctor over many years. The knowledge of the patient, who is reified, is incomplete and inaccurate. Whatever assessment the doctor makes, the knowledge of the patient is fallible and not based on an RCT. *The knowledge of the patient is different in kind from the RCT knowledge.* This surely limits the entire EBM discursive practice which projects the image that it is based on the results of clinical studies. Even so, as stated by numerous authors, the gap between the group data and the individual's suitability cannot be reduced beyond a certain, unknown, distance. *The actual susceptibility of the patient for the researched intervention cannot be precisely known.* If the clinical doctor follows the study results and invokes the intervention for her patient, we can, at best, hope and believe that that the intervention will be helpful. Regrettably, if the patient improves, we still do not *actually know* whether the intervention caused the improvement, or was coincidental.

---

[51] 1994, pp. 159-161.

2.2.7 The docile body

Foucault's *gaze* has been problematised. The trouble is that the patient does not look back! (This has been called "the docile body", and does not square with phenomenology.) There is an air of dominance here. My comments on the sufferers from AIDS are a suitable antidote. I represent these patients as active in the medical relationship.

Bloor and McIntosh noted that the subjects of the surveying therapeutic gaze responded in various ways, including direct rejection and attack on the value and legitimacy of the health worker's[52] attentions, non-cooperation, silence, escape, avoidance, and most-common of all, concealment.[53]

In my work as a Police Medical Officer, I need permission to examine every patient in police custody. Sometimes this is not granted, even when the patient asked for a doctor, and I have travelled 22 kilometers during the night. In my third year I was challenged as to whether I was a Police Medical Officer (as I had stated) or "just a doctor off the street". I always have a constable with me, so questions about the intake of drugs and aclohol, intended to help me assess the state of the brain, receive a variety of responses. Recently, in obtaining a history as to how the patient gained an incised wound in front of his patella tendon, I was given completely different accounts by the patient and constable. These police patients, then, sometimes show up one limitation of the medical gaze.

3. The medical /EBM gaze meets the smooth space of the doctor-patient consultation which includes the patient and her problems

I now bring the EBM gaze, which includes the results of epidemiological research, conducted on large groups of experimental subjects, into the smooth space of the patient. However, the reticulated knowedge of the EBM gaze is a poor fit for the smooth space of the patient. As the reticulated gaze arrives in smooth space, it leaves gaps between the laminae of the framework. Thus it fails to deal adequately with the smooth space of the patient. Consider the wild suffering and wellness that escapes medical surveillance because its flows of energy are not easily categorized into the diagnoses and tests that yield currency for EBM.

EBM has forced us to develop our understanding of the application of evidence derived from large groups of experimental subjects to the individual patient and so has addressed one of its most frequently cited problems. "The inferential leap necessary for treating an individual based on aggregate findings is mostly assumed away".[54] But in an RCT, some patients are excluded, subjects actually take their medication, the treatment period is likely to be short and closely monitored in comparison with future widespread use of the treatment, and the control condition often uses placebo treatment, not a realistic option for the "nomadic" clinician.[55] The end points of the research may differ from the outcomes of interest to the doctor and/or patient, a problem not always captured in terms of internal versus external validity.[56] The theory which the RCT provides evidence for is therefore *not*

---

[52] Strictly speaking, this quote refers to British health visitors calling on mothers, not actually to doctors.

[53] Lupton 1997, p. 104.

[54] Tanenbaum 1999, p. 757.

[55] Worrall 2010.

[56] Bluhm 2010.

the theory that the trialled treatment will, overall, be beneficial for the next patient. Therefore the relationship between group research (in striated space) and clinical care (in smooth or nomadic space) is not self-evident despite voices to the contrary.[57]

The vexed issue of how apply the findings from population research to the individual patient is partly clarified by attention to patient characteristics (including age, severity of disease, comorbidity, ethnicity, and compliance with treatment regimens), healthcare system characteristics (skills of treating doctors, treatment or test availability, monitoring) and outcome characteristics (do study outcomes matter to the present doctor/patient dyad, surrogate endpoints, such as bone density rather than fractures, and so on).[58] The clinical doctor treating the individual patient on the basis of population research needs to notice the number needed to treat figure "for a group of individuals resembling their patient",[59] and to carefully look into relative risks and absolute risks as they exist for the unselected people who walk into the clinic rather than the select group in whom study effects are seen. What is more, even though subgroup analyses reflect "patient diversity in risk for disease, responsiveness to treatment, vulnerability to adverse effects, and utility for different outcomes",[60] subgroups of one are not part of that kind of science even though they are the norm in the nomadic space of real world clinical medicine. When we add ethical considerations of patient choice and the acceptability of treatment to the mix[61] it is no wonder that results produced in a striated world do not apply at the contested margins of striation where nomadic knowledge charts its paths through smooth spaces of unstructured and sometimes chaotic experience.[62]

EBM does not tell us how to mix and match the five warrants that plausibly should attend clinical decision-making. (These are: the results of clinical research, pathophysiological reasoning, clinical experience, patient preferences and actions, and system factors {such as the availability of a test or treatment.}) Differences in ontology, methodology, epistemology and ethicality criss cross the field.[63] Firstly, there is an ontological difference between pathophysiology and system factors. For example, while pathophysiology may be anchored in the biology of antibacterials, system factors may be anchored in health economics such that a general practitioner is not allowed to prescribe certain drugs. The difference in these two warrants is ontological in that they belong to different orders of reality. Second, an epistemological difference exists between clinical experience and the results of an RCT – one depends on judgments of similarity and difference between particular instances of illness (the last spinal empyema and this one) and the other on the adequacy of inclusion and application criteria relating particular cases to a general category (this pneumonia as an

[57] Silva & Wyer 2009.
[58] Bassler, Busse, Karanicolas & Guyatt 2008.
[59] Bassler, Busse, Karanicolas & Guyatt 2008, p. 2.
[60] Bassler, Karanicolas, Busse & Guyatt 2008, p. 1.
[61] Bassler, Karanicolas, Busse & Guyatt 2008.
[62] I must admit that the frequent emphasis in my work on the chaotic nature of clinical practice is perhaps excessive, and intended to contrast with EBM. I am aware that Descartes and many other great thinkers have been struck by orderliness in the universe, and its susceptibility to mathematical modeling. And there was some structure in the clinical consultation before EBM. For example,the results of pathophysiological experiments have guided doctors for a very long time.
[63] Kerridge 2010.

instance of bacterial infection). Thirdly, there is a difference between patient preferences and and the clinical experience of the doctor as in the choice for abortion and the doctor's judgment that it will turn out badly for the woman concerned. There is a major ethical component in the way the decision is arrived at in that the patient chooses and the doctor can only advise on the basis of experience. Somehow these two warrants must be combined and how to do so is unclear.

We can draw two conclusions from this analysis of the difficulty in combining warrants for decision. One is that there is an epistemological crisis in medicine, since we now realise that we do not know how to amalgamate five streams of very different kinds of knowledge. The second is that we no longer know what (in real life) EBM is: 100 different doctors may combine the multiple warrants for decision in different ways and in this task of integrating the warrants, no schema has been agreed or even proposed.

I now direct more attention to the difficulty of combining the five warrants for decision. I actually simplify the problem by selecting just two of the five warrants. The problem then simplifies to: *how to combine the result of epidemiological research with clinical experience.* (I allow myself to wander a little between clinical experience and clinical intuition). Note that EBM uses the term "integrate" for the warrants for decision.

Deleuze and Guattari[64] provide an analysis of the impasse. (Note that there is a difference between clinical experience and clinical expertise.) Consider clinical research results and clinical expertise and recall the 2002[65] model of decision making whereby clinical expertise brokers the possibly conflicting claims of research evidence, patient preferences and actions, and clinical state and circumstances. The EBM desire to bring the results of clinical research into clinical decision making can be viewed as an attempt to striate smooth space—the epidemiological evidence is used to reticulate the smooth space of clinical experience/intuition and patient management.[66]

> *Smooth space and striated space – nomad space and sedentary space – the space in which the war machine develops and the space instituted by the state apparatus--are not of the same nature. No sooner do we note a simple opposition between the two kinds of space than we must indicate a much more complex difference by virtue of the successive terms of the oppositions fail to coincide entirely. And no sooner have we done that than we must remind ourselves that the two spaces in fact exist only in mixture: smooth space is constantly being translated, traversed into a striated space; striated space is constantly being reversed, returned to a smooth space. In the first case, one organises even the desert; in the second, the desert gains and grows; and the two can happen simultaneously. But the de facto mixes do not preclude a de jure, or abstract, distinction between the two spaces. That there is such a distinction accounts for the fact that the two spaces do not communicate with each other in the same way: it is the de jure distinction that determines the forms assumed by a given de facto mix and the direction or meaning of the mix (is a smooth space captured, enveloped by a striated space or does a striated space dissolve into a smooth space, allow a smooth space to develop?). This raises a number of simultaneous questions: the simple oppositions between the two spaces; the complex differences; the de facto mixes, and the passages from one to another; the principles of the mixture, which are not at all symmetrical,*

[64] 1987.

[65] Haynes, Devereux & Guyatt 2002.

[66] Braude 2009.

sometimes causing a passage from smooth to striated, sometimes from striated to smooth, according to entirely different movements.[67]

If this is an accurate analysis, then it follows that rational integration eludes us with regard to the desire of EBM to resolve the conflict between the results of clinical research and clinical experiences/intuition.[68]

There is another way of seeing why we cannot rationally reticulate smooth space and develop a method to overcome the difference because in the multiplicities we deal with in human life a kind of tacit knowledge, similar to clinical intuition/expertise, is indispensable.

We have on numerous occasions encountered all kinds of differences between two types of multiplicities: metric and non-metric; extensive and qualitative; centred and acentred; arborescent and rhizomatic; numerical and flat; dimensional and directional; of masses and of packs; of magnitude and of distance; of breaks and of frequency; striated and smooth.[69]

While it is possible to create rules to deal with entities that are part of the same order, it is not rationally possible to reticulate or divide up a commodity which is heterogeneous and intensive. Take pain. Although doctors ask patients to rate pain on a scale of ten, we cannot move from there to arguing that if a treatment leads a patient to change the rating of the pain intensity from 10 to five, the pain (as an orderly variable) has been halved. There are many areas of medicine not amenable to rational metrication and biostatistics because they are intrinsically relational rather than objectively fixed.

In the last few paragraphs I argue that there is no rational way to merge the results of epidemiological research with clinical intuition. I heralded an epistemological crisis in medicine, though I am not the first to do this. So what are doctors doing? The method of mixing these disparate inputs lies not in any codified system. They are joined through implicit, not explicit, knowledge, as is learned by a house surgeon from her senior. The judgments involved are learned by the less experienced doctor. Thus the epistemological crisis moves into the field of tacit knowledge. A lengthy and detailed explanation, which draws on Wittgenstein and Kuhn, of the way in which all codifiable knowledge rests in a sea of implicit knowledge is developed by Tim Thornton[70] who argues that both scientific research results and clinical expertise rest, in fact, on tacit knowledge. Whatever codified knowledge is to be used, *judgement* is required as to which codified knowledge and whether and when to use it. For example, judgment is required in selecting a theory to apply to several diverse scientific problems. Thornton points out that the best and fullest accounts of EBM make this clear, but EBM does lend itself to distortion in which evidence-*based* medicine quickly slips into codified knowledge, paying little attention to the backgound use of judgement or implicit knowledge. The devil is in the detail as to the wise use of the term "based".

If Deleuze and Guattari[71] are right, a method for reticulating decision-making warrants into evidential form is bound to fail[72] in that new forms of evidence would suffer under the

[67] Deleuze and Guattari 1987, pp. 474-475.
[68] Braude 2009.
[69] Deleuze and Guattari 1987, pp. 483-484.
[70] 2006.
[71] 1987.

tyranny of data,[73] and the whole approach of reticulating the warrants for decision into evidential form ignores the argument that the inputs cannot be construed as evidence. The attempt itself is a totalising tendency suited to a striated domain of action and not nomadic science and it marginalises the idiosyncratic aspects of patients, doctors, and their interaction so that "the movement challenges professionalism by disputing what and how physicians know, and especially by marginalising what one physician can know about one patient".[74] This encounter-based knowledge is smooth or nomadic and does not have a settled scientific home.

The assertions of EBM, focused on the importance of clinical research, falter because medicine is at the intersection of several sciences and even of diverse scholarly disciplines each with its own mode of knowing. For example, the humanities, such as anthropology and history, emphasize qualitative evidence and argument. Ethics draws heavily on rational thought and the critical examination of claims to good practice. Therefore placing evidence from epidemiology and biostatistics in the dominant position for clinical understanding is hegemonic.[75] Post-structuralist writers interweave "evidence" with issues arising when one takes note of power and regimes of truth. Misak,[76] for instance, explains that narrative evidence can provide insight into what it is like to be sick, or to receive investigation and/or treatment that is likely to escape RCTs. She gives detailed comment on how we all assess what we are told and incorporate it into our stories and provides a framework for a still better assessment of the multiplicity and richness of clinical phenomena.

4. Reflections on science in medicine

EBM attempts to put medicine on a more scientific footing, using clinical epidemiology. As is well-known, the early protagonists were concerned about variation in medical practice, cost, and the clear possiblity that even expert opinion may not square with the evidence derived from clinical research. One issue here is whether medicine can be classed as a science. The relationship between medicine and science is complex and much debated (Is medicine a science or an art? EBM protagonists have said that they will help provide the art of medicine with a scientific basis.). I take the view that medicine draws on a number of disciplines, including physiology, ethics, law, epidemiology and biostatistics, anthropology and so on. I have positioned my work to be alert to any tendency of epidemiology and biostatistics to dictate its rules of evidence to the whole of medicine. In this regard, I note that De Caro and Macarthur[77] introduce a volume which explains the difficulties scientific naturalism has in dealing with a number of issues which occur in medicine. For example, scientific naturalism, "where causes are thought of as mind-independent"[78] is under strain when it attempts to provide convincing accounts of intentional states, human freedom and personal identity, of patients, doctors and researchers. Scientific naturalism provides us with an account of objects placed in a world-as-studied-by-science. These objects can even

[72] Tanenbaum 2006.
[73] Tonelli 2007, p. 505.
[74] Tanenbaum 1999, pp. 757-758.
[75] Holmes, Murray, Perron & Rail 2006.
[76] Misak 2010.
[77] 2004.
[78] De Caro and Macarthur 2004, pp. 10-13.

include meaning, motivation and values. However, De Caro and Macarthur[79] allude to a chapter by Huw Price, which draws attention to the "metaphysically substantial conceptions of reference and truth" supporting this object world. These authors note an asymmetry in this naturalism: it is heavy on the object but light on the subject. Explaining this, De Caro and Macarthur draw attention to the negligible attention paid to use of linguistic terms and expressions. This subject naturalism is strangely omitted. There is also their tendency to accept a fundamentally foundational and exclusively true and well-ordered scheme of knowledge with a unitary structure of justification and principles of validity and worth.

I consider that epidemiology and biostatistics exemplify scientific naturalism and cannot cope adequately with some aspects (such as intentional states, freedom, personal identity) of the lives of patients. From here it is a short step (via psycho-neuro-humero-immunology) to denying epidemiology and biostatistics supreme authority in medicine. This is an example of my application of philosophy to EBM. I hope this approach savours more of providing a viewpoint than the authority of philosophy. In any event, I am comforted by the last sentence in De Caro and Macarthur's "Introduction",[80] ending..." the distinction between science and philosophy is one that is constantly being negotiated."

In further consideration of what authority science has in medicine I now provide an answer to the question I asked two paragraphs back: *Is medicine a science or an art?* Montgomery, in her book, "How doctors think",[81] tells us it is neither: it is a *practice.* By now I have argued that medicine is a practice which draws on science. If this is right we need be circumspect regarding any claim which science may make as to its authority, epistemically, in medicine. This matter has been dealt with extensively by many authors such as Miles, Loughlin and Polychronis. Rather than reiterate their viewpoints, I will limit myself to post--structuralist comment. According to Foucault, knowledge and power are inseparable. And from the point of view of Deleuze and Guattari, now that EBM has been so extensively problematised at the conceptual level by the above-mentioned authors, we are not in a position to anoint this approach to medicine as "the truth". In fact post-structuralist thinkers allow a range of pathways to knowledge, including the provision of knowledge by one doctor about one patient. Even patients can conrtibute knowledge. To what extent is the patient's pain reduced by the treatment? Heidegger, admittedly not a post-structuralist philosopher, tells us that *being* cannot be investigated as if it were an entity, using "positive" sciences like biology. Rather *being* has the struture of meaning, and is best investigated phenomenologically. It seems to me that pain is nearer to being than to an entity.

5. Conclusion

Much of what I have written has been written before. I beleive that the cutting edge of my own contribution lies in the following points. The EBM process starts in smooth space, proceeds into codified knowledge, and returns to try to striate or organise smooth space. I have highlighted the rapid distancing from the patient involved in the PICO question and I look forward to providing an existential/phenomenological account of this in a later paper

[79] 2004, p. 10.

[80] 2004, p. 17.

[81] Montgomery, K. *How doctors think. Clinical judgement and the practice of medicine.* Oxford: Oxford University Press, 2006.

on Heidegger. As the doctor assesses the suitability of the patient for the intervention she hopefully takes account of detailed advice provided by EBM leaders in 2008. Even so, I suggest that the more we focus on science, on business and on the computer, the more we move away from the relationship of yesteryear when a doctor, ideally, knew her patient. When all has been said and done, the *knowledge* which the doctor has of her patient's suitability for the intervention is of a different kind from the much-vaunted knowledge derived from clinical research. I take the view that this provides EBM with a scarcely-acknowedged soft underbelly.

I have drawn on the writings of Kerridge and Deleuze and Guattari to argue that the warrants for decision are heterogenous with reagrd to ontology, methodology, ethicality and epistemology and that they cannot be *integrated,* rationally. I have presented the process as warrants for decision being *mixed* through tacit knowledge, often learned from a senior doctor. I have presented clinical research as an example of striated space and clinical experience as an example of partly smooth space (intuition). Deleuze and Guattari explain that it is not possible to integrate smooth space and striated space. Not rationally. Thornton moves the issue into tacit knowledge.

I consider that EBM has scarcely noticed that it has partly constructed the (guidelined) doctor, the patient (consortium of variables) and the (research-infiltrated) consultation space. And it has scarcely noticed the meta-epistemological issue that it has set itself up to determine what constitutes medical knowledge and that it assumes the the visble and articulable are isomorphic. It has given no account of nomadic science and works with the belief that smooth space should be striated and that it can be striated. Never mind infinity, the smallest deviation and the space between the laminating parallel lines. EBM seems unaware that we know more than we can descibe (this relates to the way in which tacit knowledge extends beyond the explicit knowledge in which EBM trades) and that whatever does not get into the medical/EBM/gaze is not a candidate for knowledge/research.

6. References

Bassler, D., Busse, J.W., Karanicolas, P.J., & Guyatt, G.H. 'Evidence-based medicine targets the individual patient. Part 1: How clinicians can use study results to determine optimal individual care'. *ACP Journal Club,* v.148, Jun. 15 2008, pp. JC4-2.

Bassler, D., Karanicolas, P.J., Busse, J.W., & Guyatt, G.H. 'Evidence-based medicine targets the individual patient. Part 2. Guides and tools for individual decision-making'. *ACP Journal Club,* v.149, July 15 2008, pp. JC1-2.

Bluhm, R. 'Evidence-based medicine and philosophy of science.' *Journal of Evaluation in Clinical Practice,* v.16, 2010, pp. 363-364.

Braude, H.D. 'Clinical intuition versus statistics: Different modes of tacit knowledge in clinical epidemiology and evidence-based medicine.' *Theoretical Medicine and Bioethics: Philosophy of Medical Research and Practice,* published on line 23 June 2009, http://www.springerlink.com.ezproxy.otago.ac.nz/content/f60127577661t2q0/fulltext.html. Last retrieved 29/08/2010.

Canguilhem, G. *On the Normal and the Pathological.* Dordrecht, Holland / Boston, USA / London , Great Britain: D. Reidel Publishing Company, 1978.

Colebrook, C. *Understanding Deleuze.* Crows Nest, NSW, Australia: Allen and Unwin. 2002.

Coveney, J. *Food, Morals and Meaning: the pleasure and anxiety of eating.* 2nd ed, London: Routledge, 2006.

De Caro, M., & Macarthur, D. 'Introduction: The nature of naturalism'. In M. De Caro and D. Macarthur (eds) *Naturalism in Question.* Cambridge, Mass., and London, England: Harvard University Press, 2004, pp. 1-17.

Deleuze, G. *Foucault* (S. Hand & P. Bove, trans.). Minneapolis and London: University of Minnesota Press, 2006.

Deleuze, G., & Guattari, F. *A Thousand Plateaus: capitalism and schizophrenia* (B.Massumi, trans.). Minneapolis and London: University of Minnesota Press, 1987.

Foucault, M. *The Birth of the Clinic: an archaeology of medical perception.* (A. M. Sheridan Smith, Trans.). New York: Random House, 1994.

Gillett, G.R. *Bioethics in the Clinic: Hippocratic reflections.* Baltimore and London: The Johns Hopkins University Press, 2004.

Haynes, R.B., Devereaux, P.J, & Guyatt, G.H. 'Clinical expertise in the era of evidence-based medicine and patient choice'. *ACP Journal Club,* v. 136 (2), 2002, p. A11.

Holmes, D., Murray, S.J., Perron, A., & Rail, G. 'Deconstructing the evidence-based discourse in health sciences: Truth, power and fascism'. *International Journal of Evidence-based Healthcare,* v. 4, 2006, pp. 180-186.

Kerridge, I. 'Ethics and EBM: Acknowledging bias, accepting difference and embracing politics'. *Journal of Evaluation in Clinical Practice,* v.16, 2010, pp. 365-373.

Lupton, D. 'Foucault and the medicalisation critique', in Alan Petersen and Robyn Bunton (eds) *Foucault, Health and Medicine.* London and New York: Routledge, 1997, pp. 94-110.

Miles, A., Loughlin, M., & Polychronis, A. 'Evidence-based healthcare, clinical knowledge and the rise of personalised medicine'. *Journal of Evaluation in Clinical Practice,* v. 14 (5), October 2008, pp. 621-649.

Misak, C.J. 'Narrative evidence and evidence-based medicine'. *Journal of Evaluation in Clinical Practice,* v.16, 2010, pp. 392-397.

Nietzsche, F. *Thus Spoke Zarathustra: a book for everyone and nobody.* (G. Parkes, Trans.). Oxford: Oxford University Press, 2005.

Silva, S.A. & Wyer, P.C., 'Where is the wisdom? II -- Evidence-based medicine and the epistemological crisis in clinical medicine. Exposition and commentary on Djulbegovic, B., Guyatt, G.H. & Ashcroft, R.E. (2009) *Cancer Control,* 16, 158-168.' *Journal of Evaluation in Clinical Practice,* v. 15(6), 2009, pp. 899-906.

Tanenbaum, S.J. 'Evidence and Expertise: The challenge of the outcomes movement to medical professionalism'. *Academic Medicine,* v. 74 (7), 1999, pp. 757-763.

Tanenbaum, S.J. 'Evidence by any other name. Commentary on Tonelli (2006), Integrating evidence into clinical practice: an an alternative to evidence-based approaches. *Journal of Evaluation in Clinical Practice* 12, 248-256'. *Journal of Evaluation in Clinical Practice,* v.12 (3), 2006, pp. 273-276.

Tonelli, M.R. 'Advancing a casuistic model of clinical decision making: A response to commentators'. *Journal of Evaluation in Clinical Practice,* v. 13 (4), 2007, pp. 504-507.

Thornton, T. 'Tacit knowledge as the unifying factor in evidence based medicine and clinical judgement'. Online *Journal of Philosophy, Ethics and Humanities in Medicine,* March 17, 2006. Retrieved 5 April, 2011, available from http://www.peh-med.com/content/1/1/2.

Wifstad, A. 'External and internal evidence in clinical judgment: The evidence-based medicine attitude'. *Philosophy, Psychiatry & Psychology,* v.15 (2), 2008, pp. 135-139.

Worrall, J. 'Evidence: philosophy of science meets medicine.' *Journal of Evaluation in Clinical Practice,* v. 16, 2010, pp. 356-362.

5

Information Mastery – Changing the Paradigm of Patient Care with Patient-Oriented Evidence That Matters (POEM)

Shepard Hurwitz[1], David Slawson[2] and Allen Shaughnessy[3]
[1]University of North Carolina-Chapel Hill
[2]University of Virginia
[3]Allen Shaughnessy Tufts University
USA

1. Introduction

In many ways, physicians and surgeons practice in a manner reminiscent of individual care provided in the late nineteenth century. The patient presents with a complaint or condition, the physician queries the patient, gathers physical evidence from examination and other measures, performs a mental exercise that arrives

first at an answer of what the problem is, then what caused the problem then a solution (treatment) is selected from a menu of options. Though the patient presents with a problem, the approach to solving the problem was entirely driven by the education and training of the clinician. In earlier times, diagnoses and treatment were often lacking, and the role of the clinician became one of educator or comforter rather than healer.

In the early part of the 21st century more is expected of those physicians providing diagnostic and treatment services. There is a greater understanding of physiology and pathological process affecting human health, and there is a greater array of treatments for injuries and conditions. Among the contemporary patient expectations are 1) the physician is actively listening and placing the wants and needs of the patient above all else, 2) the healthcare provider is delivering the most effective means of arriving at an accurate diagnosis then providing the most appropriate care and 3) does the expected outcome of treatment meet the needs of the patient while remaining affordable. These new rules of engagement are woven into the framework of evidence-based medicine (EBM).

2. Patient centered care

EBM is patient centered, that is the patient is the center of the decision process starting with choice of diagnostic procedures, then the selection of treatment and is the evaluator of the success of treatment. Outcomes that matter to patients also matter to physicians and can be characterized as Patient Oriented Evidence that Matters (POEM). Reduction of pain, improved function, improved quality of life, reduced mortality, and reasonable cost are the cornerstone of value added to the lives of individuals who seek treatment. This might seem commonsensical and physicians traditionally think that the 19th century way of providing care has been meeting the needs outlined above. In the United States and other countries with advanced medical knowledge systems, the evidence is mounting that the needs of patients are not addressed in a patient centered way, nor are outcomes as good as physicians believe.

The fundamental process of Evidence Based-Medicine (EBM) consists of five-steps: 1) developing a question using the populations-intervention-comparison-outcome (PICO) format, 2) finding research that may answer the question, 3) evaluating the research for validity, impact, and applicability, 4) applying the information to clinical decision making, and 5) periodically evaluating one's outcomes after implementation and performance of the previous four steps.[5] The development of the question to be answered is patient centered and the EBM process focuses on issues that matter to the patient. This is a labor intense process that involves finding several sources of evidence, analyzing, evaluating and then making the product understandable by the patient.

The introduction of EBM shifted the decision making to the patient while having the physician analyze the patient within the context of evidence that is relevant to that patient and their condition. After the analysis, the diagnosis is expressed in a relativistic way using likelihood or probability to the patient in a way he or she can understand. Offering treatment is more of a menu with expected outcomes and possible unwanted outcomes freely discussed with the patient. The treatment options are based upon the highest order of evidence available, and when possible treatment guidelines based upon best evidence is given as the most reliable means to predict outcome. At times there will be good evidence to cite in the discussions with the patient, other times there will be a paucity of good evidence and the patient's decision may reflect the lack of evidence, relying more on expert opinion.

One reason physicians and surgeons rely on textbooks and content experts is the time factor. It is very easy and quick to call a colleague for an opinion or formally consult a colleague for either input on evaluation or treatment- or to assume care of a challenging patient problem. When clinicians do spend their time searching for answers to questions or problems, the easiest sources are textbooks, review articles, audio reproductions of lectures and information provided by pharmaceutical and implant companies. Again, easy location of didactic information consumes less time and energy than a thorough search and analysis of possibly relevant, possibly useful information.

Clinicians develop idiosyncratic ways of evaluating, communicating and interacting with their patients- often a direct reflection of residency/fellowship training. One tactic is not providing answers to patient's questions or questions of care, probably due to a combination of factors- lack of time and little knowledge. Many feel that by reading current literature and attending CME courses that they are indeed keeping up with meaningful change and offering their patients the best practice based upon the best current knowledge. The clinician's sense of security by maintaining exposure to relevant topics in the literature is a culture of habit- reading familiar journal articles, reliance on consultants, compliance with local customs or referral patterns and reliance on quick sources of information- textbooks, review articles, electronic media, colleagues etc. While these sources may be of great value, there is a high probability that they are out of date or biased. One of the most ingrained biases in all medical literature is the highly selective patient population described in texts and manuscripts- often the idealized patient in a study is not very similar to the patient in the doctor's practice, or the real world patient has multiple problems while the textbook discusses only one problem at a time.

Decision-making is another key element of evidence based medicine. There is the continual need to remind ourselves that patient care is about patients making decisions that affect outcome. The earlier notion of shared decision making has now shifted with the EBM paradigm to patient-centered decision making. The physician is once again a 'doctor'- from the Latin 'teacher'.

3. Sources of evidence

There are three main sources of medical information that can be used in generating evidence. First is primary sources material. This is the collection of original publications that answer questions about patient care. Next are the review articles, textbooks, synopses and curriculum of courses that are the first attempt to synthesize evidence with opinions. Most of the teaching at the Medical School level is in this second level, as are the popular texts and review courses. Third is the assimilation of best evidence via systematic reviews, meta-analysis and generation of evaluation or treatment guidelines.

The first level of primary source is the substrate that is entered into the evidence production cycle. The production cycle creates evidence in response to a clinical need, refines the results of investigations to craft an answer to the question raised by the clinical need. Once meaning is added to the data gathered, this evidence is now disseminated via publications or presentations, the evidence is put into practice and lastly the evidence is evaluated to determine if further evidence is needed to better solve the original need. The role of generating evidence is fundamental, however, the need for dissemination and implementation become almost as important if the evidence is to be used to improve quality of care.

The second level of information is the synthesis of opinions and creation of literature that informs clinicians about what is available. This group includes review articles, textbooks, online texts and review lectures. As a source of evidence, this second level is highly variable in that expert opinion may supersede the synthesis of the best evidence, and other bias may creep into the review product. The third level is the combination of best evidence with critical analysis provided by experts in methods of providing statistical support for best evidence. These are the systematic reviews of evidence and meta-analysis. Studies that combine first level evidence into stronger support statements, or non-support statements of diagnostic and treatment evidence.

Medical knowledge is stratified in a pyramidal formula created by Bloom in the 1950s (see figure 1). Recall or remembering is the entry level of knowledge with understanding and applying the next two levels that are necessary in medical practice. Most clinicians operate mostly in the first three levels of knowledge and rely on sources than can analyze, evaluate and create the understanding and application for improving medical knowledge. This taxonomy of learning is similar to the creation of best evidence and application to patient care.

The importance again of disseminating the evidence is essential for improving quality of care, and later on an evaluation of care after implementation is needed to determine if more and better evidence is still needed.

4. Information mastery

EBM has created several concepts and principles that are embodied in "a hierarchy of evidence and that conclusions related to evidence from controlled experiments are accorded

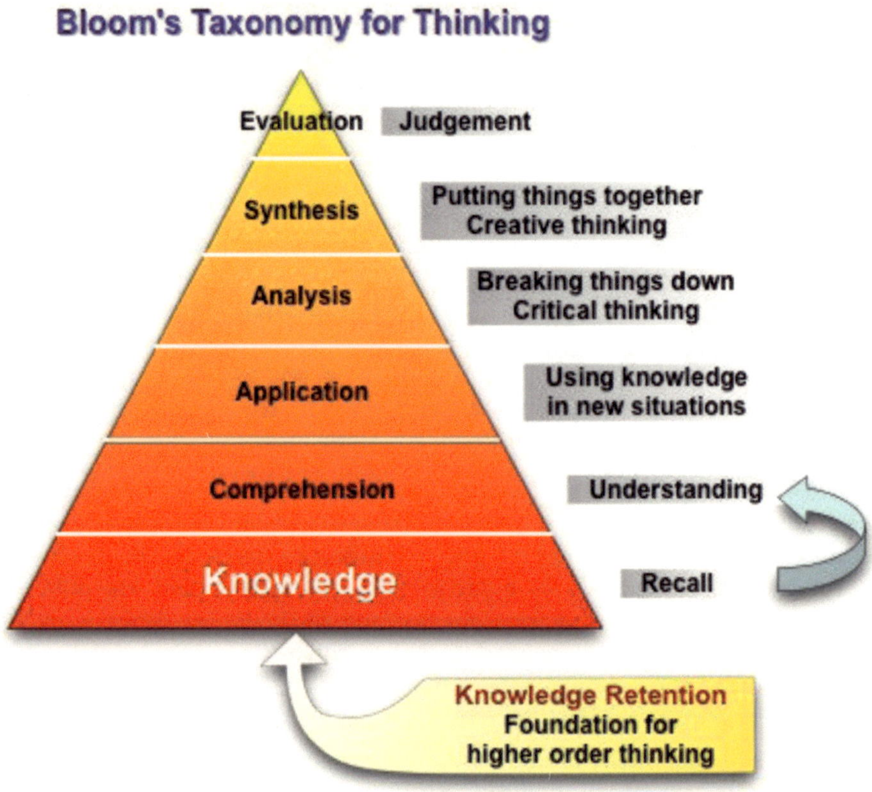

(University of Texas, Arlington, Center for Learning accessed via Google, 10/21.2011)

Fig. 1.

greater credibility than conclusions grounded in other sorts of evidence." In this hierarchy there is a (unproven) belief by advocates of EBM that randomized control trials- the highest level of evidence- should trump evidence from non-randomized trials and case-comparison studies. The lowest levels of evidence consist of case series and expert opinion. Though logical, there remains a great deal of reluctance on the part of practicing physicians to abandon their comfort zone in the reliance on expert opinion and studies that do not use comparative cohorts of patients. And the unaddressed problem of relevance, that is most studies do not include the complexity seen in most 'real world' patients.

5. The usefulness of evidence

With the advent of new and better evidence have come guidelines based upon evidence. Having guidelines is a shortcut for doctors who can follow key elements of evidence-based practice without having to do extensive literature research and analyses. This is one of the fundamental principles of information mastery- the usefulness principle, expressed as an equation:

$$\text{Usefulness} = \text{Relevance x Validity/ Work}$$

Where **relevance** is the similarity of the real world patient to that portrayed in the guideline and general applicability of the evidence, **validity** is the scientific truthfulness of the information and **work** is the amount of time spent finding the answer to a question in clinical diagnosis or treatment. Validity is of prime importance with relevance a close second.

Simply stated, the Usefulness Equation is a form of Occam's Razor- finding the simplest solution to a problem with the important features of the process being 1) likelihood of success and 2) ease of access to the information needed to make judgments and decisions. This is not a quantitative equation but gives a sense of the relationship between the key elements of best evidence.

Learning mastery is a means of educating students in a linear fashion. Students are taught basics or fundamentals, and then they are shown how to apply process to the fundamentals to solve problems and create higher cognitive functioning. An example is learning numbers and then learning to make sentences with numbers- i.e. equations- applying addition, subtraction etc. Similar to learning mastery is information mastery. A process in which adult learners are instructed in basic functions about finding information that is used to solve problems and answer questions. An example is using the Internet to search for the best treatment of a 40-year-old woman who smokes, has a BMI of 34 and presents with pneumonia. With the patient care issue, the best use of the internet is not to have a search engine deliver thousands of journal articles that would take countless hours and a great deal of analytic skill to synthesize a treatment. The Internet can now provide rapid access to treatment guidelines, protocols and algorithm based upon high level of evidence that will produce good outcomes at reasonable cost, if the patient agrees with the recommended treatment.

With the advent of information technology and the availability of sources of reliable evidence vetted by experts in the EBM it is now feasible to instruct clinicians in where to find and how to implement usable best evidence. Rather than frustrate busy practitioners with the laborious process of generating their own best evidence, the time is best spent gathering evidence and EBM guidelines.

Slawson and Shaugnessy (2003) have created and tested a curriculum to teach the principles of information management. The curriculum has three levels:

- Level 1 is for clinicians who can use the concepts to make better patient-care decision;
- Level 2 is for teachers and writers who teach clinicians the curriculum and provide evidence-based reviews of original research; and
- Level 3 is for researchers who are adept at conducting decision analysis, meta-analysis, and other techniques of synthesizing raw research information into useable clinical information.

6. Locating information from available sources

Finding the information at the point of care (just in time) is at the core of how the application of evidence-based medicine can transform the practice of medicine in ways that save time, cost, suffering and lives. The combination of clinical and laboratory diagnosis with the technology to bring validated treatment plans into use makes for less reliance on the doctor's memory or experience. Given the current focus on patient safety and reducing medical diagnostic and treatment errors, there is great advantage to putting systems-based solutions in place that override the individual decision making of physicians. With evidence-based medicine, there is no need for doctors to memorize and catalogue volumes of information 'just in case' they need it. There now exists 'just in time' information that is processed into usable guidelines that inform and educate the patient while providing a more reliable process that protects patient safety and delivers better outcomes.

There are two 'tools' in information mastery that apply to 'just in time' application of evidence at the point of care. First are hunting tools, second are foraging tools (figure 2).

A high-quality foraging tool employs a transparent process that:

1. filters out disease-oriented research and presents only patient-oriented research outcomes,
2. demonstrates that a validity assessment has been performed using appropriate criteria,
3. assigns levels of evidence, based on appropriate validity criteria, to individual studies,
4. provides specific recommendations, when feasible, on how to apply the information, placing it into clinical context,
5. comprehensively reviews the literature for a specific specialty or discipline, and
6. coordinates with a high-quality hunting tool.

A high-quality hunting tool employs a transparent process that:

1. uses a specific, explicit method for comprehensively searching the literature to find relevant and valid information,
2. provides key recommendations supported by patient oriented outcomes when possible, and, when not, specified as preliminary when supported only by disease-oriented outcomes,
3. assigns levels of evidence+ or strength of recommendation# to key recommendations using approved criteria,
4. coordinates with a reliable foraging tool.

(Ebell, 2003)

Fig. 2. Criteria for High-Quality Hunting and Foraging Tools

Hunting tools are information resources that have already organized the literature-based information by relevance, having synthesized the validity into a product that can be easily (quickly) accessed by electronic search media. There is a simple rating system for the combined validity and relevance called the Strength of Recommendation Taxonomy (SORT). The importance of a combined system such as SORT is that it meets the conditions of the Usefulness Equation- it is easy to locate (low work) and has high relevance and validity. An additional quality that is of value in a hunting tool is the transparency displayed. The issues surrounding transparency include the description of the process used in the generation of evidence as well as conflicts of interest with stakeholders in the results of the evidence. Though many physicians are capable of their interpretation and analysis of medical literature, including relevance and validity, it is time consuming and impractical to do this on a regular basis. Once again the Usefulness Equation discourages intensive searching or analytics because of the work involved. Perhaps such analysis and discovery is useful for clinical research but is unwieldy for patient care. The ideal source for best evidence should be independent of bias, thoroughly searches the literature, expertly assesses the validity and then summarizes the content in a concise, readable outline for the reader.

In addition to hunting tools that zoom-in on the relevance and validity, are the second major type of location tools- foraging. These are sources that have valid information that helps the clinician keep current. Newer patient-oriented evidence may be published but unless the clinician knows of the existence of such newer knowledge, the physician does not know that there is a need to change practice. The incorporation of foraging tools into clinical does not require point of care application but is part of the background work that should be done by those assuming patient care responsibility. As with the hunting tools, these foraging tools are transparent, explaining methods, criteria for entry and exclusion and outlining conflicts of interest among stakeholders. The habitual use of a foraging tool prompts the clinician of patient oriented evidence that will keep practice current; however some review of the relevance and validity of these sources is needed before adopting recommendations. Unlike hunting tools, the practitioner is not looking for clinical pathways or immediate answers to patient care questions.

Relevance is the patient-centered aspect of EBM. The evidence that helps with patients making decisions is identifying patient-oriented evidence that matters (POEM). This POEM matters to the clinician as well and is what physicians and surgeons should be searching for and present to their patients for consumption prior to decisions.

Three questions that help assess the evidence as POEM:

5. Did the study or guideline evaluate an outcome, and is the outcome one that patients care about?
6. Did the study or guideline evaluate a condition, disease or issue that is congruent with patients in your practice?
7. If the evidence is true, would the discovery of that truth require you to incorporate this finding into your practice?

Validity is the most scientifically and intellectually challenging element of evidence based medicine. Analysis and assessment of information that is considered evidence is difficult and time consuming. For those without the background needed to dissect methodology, statistical plans, bias, accuracy and error- it is most difficult to arrive at a judgment about the validity of any medical research. And if the outcome is a disease status or a surrogate endpoint for what matters to most patients, it is an even more difficult challenge. Having reliable hunting and foraging tools brings the world of evidence back into the realm of patient care for the majority of clinicians who do not have the training, inclination or time to apply scientific rigor to patient care information. Again, some level of assessment of the relevance is needed in conjunction with validity in order to satisfy the Usefulness Equation.

Information that is not valid is not useful, and information that is not relevant is not useful. If the amount of work to find evidence is excessive, the clinician will not consistently put that amount of effort into the process. Other sources of information become the default search engine- textbooks, review articles etc.

Value in healthcare is currently defined as an equation:

$$\text{Value} = \text{Quality} / \text{Cost}$$

Quality is the desired outcome of treatment while cost is monetary amount needed to provide treatment. Cost includes the added expense of treating complications, errors and poor results, plus the loss in earnings and savings required to pay for services. Providing improved quality increases value, as does decreasing cost. The potential for EBM and guidelines is the improvement in quality- by bringing the delivery of an outcome that is closer to the expectation of the patient the quality metric improves. There is evidence now that improved quality, by reducing unwanted outcomes and complications, will reduce cost. Thus a more robust increase in value is created if both the numerator and the denominator of the Value Equation can be properly affected.

7. Summary

A great deal has been written and taught about patient-centered decision making and patient centered care. The shift from expert opinion and experience-based learning toward best evidence and clinical practice guidelines is a shift in our medical learning and practice. Critical evaluation of patient care requires a metric that is based on outcome, which in turn requires reflection by the physician on how well the diagnoses and treatments are working in a given patient population. There is value to learning from one's practice- that is now considered a core competency in residency training in the United States. The improvement in patient outcomes that is expected with newer medical knowledge is, in itself, a delivery system of evidence to the point of care. Familiarity with sources of best evidence and practice guidelines is a reasonable next step to improve upon historical performance of physicians and surgeons. Reducing errors & complications, improving compliance with best practice, lowering costs, meeting patient expectations are lofty goals that require a newer way of problem solving than that of the past century. Tools exist for finding best evidence quickly and content experts have already done the heavy lifting by gathering and analyzing the primary sources, creating tertiary sources of good evidence. Though high-level evidence does not yet exist in many areas of clinical practice, there is ample evidence that could be put into practice now. Using available information sources and experience, information mastery facilitates putting that which is better into practice and will create evidence-based, patient centered care.

8. References

[1] ACGME Outcomes Project, General competencies http://www.acgme.org/outcome/comp/compFull.asp Accessed 12 November 2009.

[2] Slawson, D.C., Shaugnessy, A.F.: Teaching Evidence Based Medicine: Should We Be Teaching Information Management Instead? Academic Medicine 80: 685-689, 2005

[3] Menzel, H. Sociological perspectives on the information-gathering practices of the scientific investigator and the medical practitioner. In: McCord D (ed). Bibliotheca Medica: Physician for Tomorrow. Boston: Harvard Medical School, 1966: 127-28.

[4] Committee on Quality Health Care in American, Institute of Medicine. Crossing the Quality Chasm: A New Health System for The 21st Century. Washington, DC: National Academy Press, 2001: 5-6.

[5] Sackett DL, Straus SE, Richardson WS, Rosenberg W, Haynes RB. Evidence-Based Medicine. How to Practice and Teach EBM. New York: Churchill Livingstone, 2000, 3-6.

[6] Shaughnessy AF, Slawson DC, Bennett JH. Becoming an information master: a guidebook to the medical information jungle. J Fam Pract. 1994; 39:489-99.
[7] Grad R, Macaulay AC, Warner M. Teaching evidence-based medical care: description and evaluation. Fam Med. 2001; 33:602-6.
[8] Schilling LM, Steiner JF, Lundahl K, Anderson RJ. Residents' patient-specific clinical questions: opportunities for evidence-based learning. Acad Med. 2005; 80:51-56.
[9] Simon HA. Models of Man, Social and Rational: Mathematical Essays on Rational Human Behavior in a Social Setting. New York: Wiley, 1957.
[10] Carter BS, Leuthner S. Decision making in the NICU – strategies, statistics and "satisficing". Bioethics Forum. 2002; 18:7-15.
[11] Gigernenzer G, Todd PM. Simple Heuristics that Make Us Smart. New York: Oxford University Press, 1999.
[12] Green ML, Ciampi MA, Ellis PJ. Residents' medical information needs in clinic: are they being met? Am J Med. 2000; 109:218-23.
[13] Riordan FAI, Boyle EM, Phillips B. Best paediatric evidence: is it accessible and used on-call? Arch Dis Child. 2004; 89:469-71.
[14] McColl A, Smith H, White P, Field J. General practitioners' perceptions of the route to evidence-based medicine: a questionnaire survey. BMJ. 1998; 316:361-65.
[15] Putnam, W, Twohig PL, Burge FI, Jackson LA, Cox JL. A qualitative study of evidence in primary care: what the practitioners are saying. CMAJ. 2002; 166:1525-30.
[16] Sackett DL, Straus SE. Finding and applying evidence during clinical rounds: the "evidence cart". JAMA. 1998; 280:1336-38.
[17] Sloane PA, Brazier H, Murphy AW, Collins T. Evidence based medicine in clinical practice: how to advise patients on the influence of age on outcome of surgical anterior cruciate ligament reconstruction: a review of the literature. Br J Sports Med. 2002; 36:200-3.
[18] Oxman AD, Sackett DL, Guyatt GH. Users' guides to the medical literature. I. How to get started. JAMA. 1993; 270:2093-95.
[19] Schulz KF, Chalmers I, Hayes RJ, et al. Subverting randomization in controlled trials. JAMA. 1995; 273:408-12.
[20] Schulz, KF, Grimes DA. Allocation concealment in randomized trials: defending against deciphering. Lancet. 2002; 359:614-18.
[21] Ebell MH, Siwek J, Weiss BD, et al. Strength of recommendation taxonomy (SORT): a patient-centered approach to grading evidence in the medical literature. Am Fam Physician. 2004; 69:548-56.
[22] Shaughnessy AF, Slawson DC, Bennett JH. Becoming an information master: a guidebook to the medical information jungle. J Fam Pract. 1994; 39:489-99.
[23] Green ML, Ciampi MA, Ellis PJ. Residents' medical information needs in clinic: are they being met? Am J Med. 2000; 109:218-23.
[24] Ely JW, Osheroff JA, Ebell MH, et al. Analysis of questions asked by family doctors regarding patient care. BMJ. 1999; 319:358-61.
[25] Ebell MH, Shaughnessy AF. Information mastery: integrating continuing medical education with the information needs of clinicians. J Cont Ed Health Prof. 2003; 23:S53-62.
[26] Shaughnessy AF, Slawson DC. Are we providing doctors with the training and tools for lifelong learning? BMJ 1999; 13:1280. pdf>. Accessed 9 April 2005.
[27] InfoPOEMs, Inc. home page http://www.InfoPOEMs.com/. Accessed 18 November 2009.
[28] JournalWatch Online http://www.jwatch.org/. Accessed 18 November 2009.

[29] Dynamed home page http://www.dynamicmedical.com. Accessed 29 November 2009.
[30] Helwig AL, Flynn D. Using palmtop computers to improve students' evidence-based decision making. Acad Med. 1998; 73:603-4.
[31] Leung GM, Johnston JM, Tin KYK, et al. A cluster randomized trial of clinical decision support tools to improve evidence-based medicine learning in medical students. BMJ. 2003; 327:1090.
[32] Johnston JM, Leung, GM, Tin KYK, et al. Evaluation of handheld clinical decision support tool for evidence-based learning and practice in medical undergraduates. Med Educ. 2004; 38:628-37.
[33] Shaughnessy AF, Schlicht JR, Vanscoy GJ, Merenstein JH. Survey and evaluation of newsletters marketed to family physicians. J Am Board Fam Pract. 1992; 5:573-79.
[34] Slawson DC, Shaughnessy AF, Barry J. Which should come first: rigor or relevance? J Fam Pract. 2001; 50:209-10.
[35] Shaughnessy AF, Slawson DC. What happened to the valid POEMs? A survey of review articles on the treatment of type 2 diabetes. BMI. 2003; 327:266-69.
[36] Slawson DC, Shaughnessy AF. Teaching information mastery: creating informed consumers of medical information. J Am Board Fam Pract. 1999. 12:444-49.
[37] Rosser WW, Slawson DC, Shaughnessy AF. Information Mastery: Evidence-Based Family Medicine. 2nd ed. Hamilton, Ontario, BC: Decker Inc., 2004.
[38] Center for Information Mastery, University of Virginia http://www.healthsystem.virginia.edu/internet/familymed/docs/info_mastery.cfm. Accessed 18 November 2009.
[39] InfoPOEMs, Inc. Events. http://www.infopoems.com/events.cfm. Accessed 18 November 2009.
[40] American Board of Medical Specialties Maintenance of Certification http://www.abms.org/MOC.asp. Accessed 18 November 2009.
[41] Smith R. What information do doctors need? BMJ. 1996; 313:1062-67.
[42] Chueh H, Barnett GO. "Just-in-time" clinical information. Acad Med. 1997; 72:512-17.
[43] Cassel EJ. The nature of suffering and the goals of medicine. N Engl J Med. 1982; 306:639-45.
[44] Cassel EJ. Diagnosing suffering: a perspective. Ann Intern Med. 1999; 131:531-34.
[45] Steward M, Brown JB, Weston WW, et al. Patient-Centered Medicine. Transforming the Clinical Method. Thousand Oaks, CA: Sage Publications, 1995.
[46] Curley SP, Yates JF, Young MJ. Seeking and applying diagnostic information in a health care setting. Acta Psychol (Amst). 1990; 73:211-23.
[47] Curley SP, Connelly DP, Rich ED. Physicians' use of medical knowledge resources: preliminary theoretical framework and findings. Med Decis Making. 1990; 10:231-41.
[48] Schon DA. The Reflective Practitioner. How Professionals Think in Action. New York: Basic Books, 1983: 42.
[49] Hurwitz, S.R., Slawson, D. A., Shaughnessy, A.: Orthopaedic Information Mastery: Applying Evidence- Based Information Tools to Improve Patient Outcome While Saving Orthopaedists' Time. Journal of Bone Joint Surgery. 2000; 82A: 888-895.
[50] Orthopaedic Web Links www.orthopaedicweblinks.com/news. Accessed 30 November 2009
[51] Banzi R.,, Liberati A., Moschetti I., Tagliabue L., Moja L.: A Review of Online Evidence-Based Practice Point-of-Care Information Summary Providers. J Med Internet Res. 2010; 12:26-39.
[52] Hurwitz SR., Slawson DC.: Should We Be Teaching Information Management Instead of Evidence-Based Medicine? Clin Orthop Rel Res. 2010;468:2633-2639.

6

Evidence Based Information Prescription (IPs) in Developing Countries

Vahideh Zarea Gavgani
Department of Medical Library & Information Science, Tabriz University of Medical Sciences, Tabriz, Iran

1. Introduction

Information Prescription (IPs) is provision of specific evidence based health information to a specific individual/patient to help him/her understand, manage and control the ill health. Most of the time it is defined as prescription of right information to right person at right time (Kemper-Mettler, 2002a). Maybe this definition is the simplest way for describing a powerful complex process. To borderline the right person at right time and offer the right information at right time in practice is really huge work. Information prescription pledge active participation of patient in healthcare process. It promises that information intervention may boost the healthcare outcomes, reduce the medical errors and undertake the patients' right. But we need to clearly illustrate it in our practice. How information therapy and information prescription can boost health care, what is the differences between patient education and information prescription? How a piece of evidence based information can be given to a patient who should make decision about her\his health in an emergency condition? Is it really possible in practice? The philosophy of Ix and prescription of information to patient is perfect. It brings patient in the field and gives a colorful sense to patient centered healthcare. What is significant in this process is that every environment has its own norms, condition, beliefs, communication style and language, social and cultural features that influence in practicing Information therapy (Ix). IIt is essential to put information therapy into practice to find out an applicable model for a specific environment. Through this pilot model, appropriate protocols and guidelines can be developed to reach the best practice. Fulfillment of IPs relies on, at least, three components i.e. Information Technology (IT), Patients Preference and Physicians Interest. IT manifestations like Internet, social networking tools, mobile phone/computer facilities are widely available for patients and physicians equally, in developed countries. In such IT based environment patients are either seeking health information or have access to the net to communicate with their physicians, receive IPs, search for health information and share their story and information with their networks. In consequence, Information Prescriptions is now part of healthcare system of developed counties like US and UK.

2. Our current status where Ix and IP to be practiced

In Iran, as a sample of a developing country, almost 100% of patients demand for information prescription and information therapy service offered by hospital or the physician who offer healthcare services to them (Gavgani, 2011). Fortunately 97% of clinical specialists believe that patients have right to information therapy services and information prescription need to be given to patients as part of their healthcare service (Gavgani,2010-2011). Access to the internet is available for individuals and professionals through ADSL and Dial UP services. The speed is limited to 64MBPS, 128 mbps higher for individual and professional. According to NetIndex the average download speed in Iran is 0.48mbps and higher in ranking the downloading speed of countries Iran ranks 167th among 168 countries (AsrIran,2011). Not all people afford high speed and unlimited internet access. The majority of ordinary internet users utilize 64 and 128 mbps speed internet access. All people do not have a computer to connect to the Internet, not all physicians uses computer with web in their office. Patients in Iran prefer to receive information therapy services in print format and most preferably in person from their health providers rather than Internet and library. However, mobile phone is also one of the most used devices by people for communication and transferring information therefore it also is a preferable device for delivering IPs to patients in Iran. Patients demand for information about diseases, treatments and medications (Gavgani, 2011). According to the above mentioned facts we had to adopt information therapy standards and guidelines to generate and develop an information therapy model applicable to our present situation with specific barriers that we face. We decided practice Information Therapy and Information Prescription for a limited subject area as a pilot project to find out the potentials, barriers, and driver forces in a model applicable for our social and cultural condition.

The main Objective of this project was provision of IPs for patients with cardiovascular problems, hospitalized in Shahid Madani Cardiology Hospital (Tabriz-Iran)from November 2011 to February 2011 ,during four months . It also aimed to detect the barriers and requirements for filling IPs in non-wired condition and reach to a sustainable and applicable model for fulfillment of IPs in developing and non-wired countries.

3. Preparing data base for information therapy and information prescription

Cardiovascular system and cardiac diseases includes a broad subject area especially it doubles when the other diseases interconnect with them. To identify the information services coverage we limited our service area to only coronary artery diseases (CAD). At first we extracted MeSH tree term map for CAD from MeSH data base (http://www.ncbi.nlm.nih.gov/mesh) [Figure1]. It enabled us to manage our information retrieval and storing model.

CAD in relation with coronary disease	CAD in Relation with Arteriosclerosis	Cad in relation with Vascular disease
Coronary Artery Disease BT:Cardiovascular Diseases BT: Heart Diseases BT: Myocardial Ischemia BT: Coronary Disease	Coronary Artery Disease BT: Arteriosclerosis BT: Arterial Occlusive Diseases BT:Vascular Diseases BT:Cardiovascular Diseases	Coronary Artery Disease [C14.907.585.250.260] BT:Coronary Disease BT:Myocardial Ischemia BT: Vascular Diseases BT: Cardiovascular Diseases BT: Diseases Category

Fig. 1. Relation between CAD and other subjects according to MeSH

According to the MeSH the broader terms /subjects for CAD can be recognized in coronary diseases, myocardial Ischemia, among heart disease. It also can be related to Arteriosclerosis, Arterial Occlusive Diseases and cardiovascular diseases. Therefore we prepared evidence based patient information for all the above mentioned three categories. Figure 2 presents tree numbers and entry terms in MeSH data base.

National Library of Medicine - Medical Subject Headings

2011 MeSH

MeSH Descriptor Data

Return to Entry Page

Standard View. Go to Concept View; Go to Expanded Concept View

MeSH Heading	Coronary Artery Disease
Tree Number	C14.280.647.250.260
Tree Number	C14.907.137.126.339
Tree Number	C14.907.585.250.260
Scope Note	Pathological processes of CORONARY ARTERIES that may derive from a congenital abnormality, atherosclerotic, or non-atherosclerotic cause.
Entry Term	Arteriosclerosis, Coronary
Entry Term	Atherosclerosis, Coronary
Entry Term	Coronary Arteriosclerosis
Entry Term	Coronary Atherosclerosis
See Also	Atherectomy, Coronary
Allowable Qualifiers	BL CF CI CL CN CO DH DI DT EC EH EM EN EP ET GE HI IM ME MI MO NU PA PC PP PS PX RA RH RI RT SU TH UR US VE VI
Entry Version	CORONARY ARTERY DIS
Previous Indexing	Coronary Disease (1966-1986)
History Note	2008 (1987); for CORONARY ARTERIOSCLEROSIS use CORONARY DISEASE 1974-1986; for CORONARY ARTERY DISEASE use CORONARY DISEASE

Fig. 2. Coronary Disease in MeSH tree

We extracted information from accurate resources including Cochrane library (www.cochrane.org), Medline Plus (www.nlm.nih.gov/medlineplus), MD Consult (www.mdconsult.com), RxList (www.rxlist.com/), Kaiser permanent (www.kaiserpermanente.org), Mayo Clinic (www.mayoclinic.com) and Pubmed clinical queries (http://www.ncbi.nlm.nih.gov/pubmed/clinical). According to Iranian nations cultural and religious background we also extracted description of a healthy heart from Holy Quran (http://www.parquran.com) and religious sources to use as standard for patient. We categorized information into three 1) Disease related health information: included information about diseases most of the time background information about Myocardial Infarction (MI), Myocardial Ischemia, Blood Pressure, Diabetics and in association with MI , Kidney Failure in relation with MI and so on. 2) Diagnostic information like Angiography. 3) Information for intervention which itself divided into two subcategories surgery, plus subcategories i.e. before and after operation, Angioplasty, CABG; and drug intervention such as Warfarin, Plavix, Aspirin, interaction and side effects of drugs. Our information prescriptions for after operational healthcare control and management of diseases was a little bit different information according to cultural and religious background of society. There are rich sources of Islamic rules in Quran (www.parsquran.com) and hadiths (saying) (http://www.tebyan.net/index.aspx?pid=65874;) for sexual relationship, mental health and nutrition therefore unlimited relationships and alcohol were not cause and concern for these society. Instead concerns around performing prayer, sympathy and being deep imaginative in sorrowful incidents with religious root were negotiable. We prepared information on when to start exercise and sexual relationship, what kind of exercise and heavy works they can or can't do, how important is taking medicine on time and in a regular style for their recovery and disease control. We also included the side effects of eating much and bad eating style, time of and number of taking meal per day, some foods and activities according to Islamic rules and Quran. After extracting and collecting data we added value to information according to library science rules (Gavgani, 2009; 2011). Information translated into Persian , simplified and made readable with 6 and 7 grade. Then We used dicsern (www.dicsern.org.uk) questionnaire's criteria to build the structure of IPs and also Ix standards using Ix standards (Kemper-Mettler, 2002b). Finally, we stored information in simple database.

4. Practice of Information Prescription (IPs) services

We asked specialists whether they would like to practice information therapy and evidence based information prescription in a team work with information specialists. Two cardiologists accepted to work with us in information therapy and to prescribe information for their patients. Then we joined to the ward round as a team member, we noted down the problems while cardiologists were taking history, explaining the case to their assistants (residents). Physicians according to the hospitals traditional method used to give brief oral information to patients during the visit and history taking. But in this project despite of the traditional model cardiologists ordered personalized information for each case that is called information prescription when needed. It means that all information were not applicable for all patients in the ICU. For example a 36 year married man who had been operated with stent placement , and had drug addiction, smoking cigarette was prescribed information about Angioplasty, stent placement, drug, smoke and exercise. We prepared the information from the small database that we had made ready already, personalized it and submitted to the cardiologist, he approved information and one of the assistants offered information to the patient and explained it once orally to patient. Patient requested instruction for *sexual* relationship information. That is ordered again by assistant to our information team. We again extracted and personalized it and gave to specialist to approve or reject it.

The other case was a 60 year old woman with 90kg weight who was accepted with heart attack and arrhythmia. She was also in inset of diabetics. She was prescribed information about pacemaker batteries, diet and lowering the weight, being alerted about airtime, sugar and LDL , HDL level, the risk of being diabetic and its relation with MI and heart attack. During taking history she said she can never go on diet because she is crazy of delicious foods with oil and sweets. We offered her extra information about Islamic instructions on eating style, quantity and time of taking food. Especially we stressed on the Islamic recommendation on "stop eating before you feel full".

A common model we used in our information prescription and information therapy service scenario is documented in a flowchart [Figure 3]. However it is significant to note that the process can be practiced with some differences according to the type of disease and patient's moment in care.

In some cases the only recommendation to patient is to repeat/to follow the previous instructions in such situation there would not be IP order therefore process will end with no need IP as shown in figure 3.

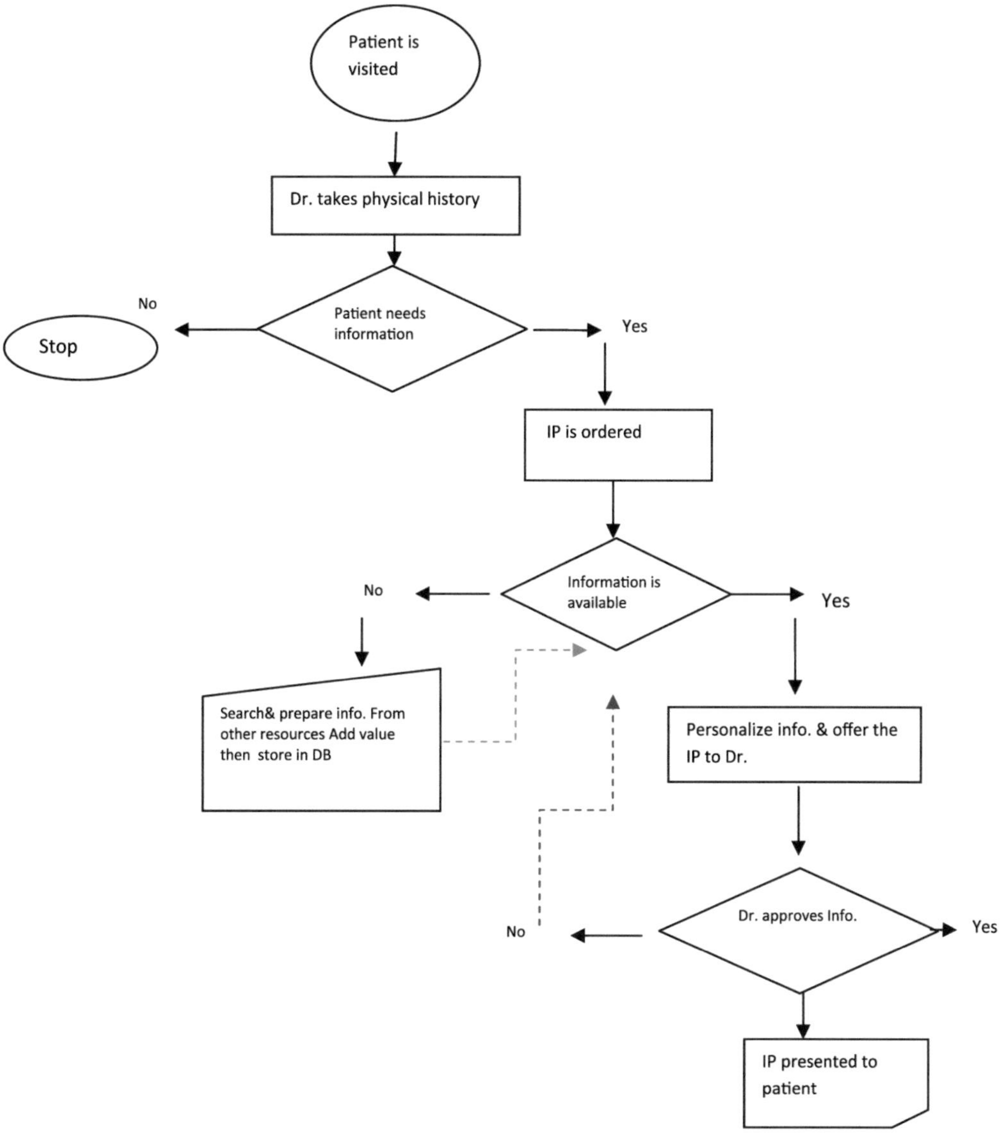

Fig. 3. The process of IP service in this project (flowchart)

5. Result

About 1500 patients with coronary Artery Disease (CAD) accepted in Shahid Madani Hospital during the months October to February 2010. The prescription were given only to those who candidate for state placement and were in professional relation with our two cardiologists. Total number of patients received IPs was 95. The average age of patients was 37.5. The youngest age was 34 and the oldest was 75. Major topics of IPs related to the Coronary Artery Disease (CAD) classified into four main categories including: diagnosis, treatment, surgery, medicine (Table 3).

Diagnosis	Treatment	Surgery	Medicine	General
Coronary Angiography	Therapeutic Lifestyle Changes (TLC) -Diet ---Dietary Approaches to Stop Hypertension (DASH) -Exercise -Weight control	Angioplasty	Effient	CAD
Cardiac Catheterization	Percutaneous Coronary Intervention (PCI)	Stent placement	Aspirin	Other

Table 3. category of prescription given to the patients with CAD

The causes of CAD can be affected by different factors such as atherosclerosis, heart attack (angina), arrhythmia, sudden cardiac arrest (SCA), heart failure, diabetes , high blood pressure, high blood cholesterol. But in this study we excluded the causes and only included IPs related to the four above mentioned main categories, plus a category named "General" about CAD and other topics. The subcategory "other" includes information which was offered to patients by doctor's demand for specific cases or patients' request such as high blood pressure (HB), Sexual relations, Addiction, MI, religious recommendations and so on.

Diagnosis	F (%)	Surgery	F (%)	Medicine	F (%)	Treatment*	F (%)	General	F (%)
Angiography	50 (82%)	Angioplasty	95 (50%)	Effient	94 (98%)	TCI	169 (97.7%)	CAD	95 (55.9%)
Catheterization	11 (18%)	Stent	95 (50%)	Aspirin	2 (2%)	PCI	4 (2.3%)	other	75 (41%)
Total	61 (8.9%)		190 (27.5 %)		96 (14%)		173 (25%)		170 (24.6%)
N= 690									

*we separated the category of medicines from treatment and divided the category of treatment into PCI and TCI . Indeed, this study has taken place in heat surgery department not internal heart disease. Therefore, the two above mentioned medicines are only medications that usually are prescribed for patients after heart surgery. About other medications like infection control medicine we did not have IP order.

Table 4. Information offered for patients through their IP order

CAD, Angioplasty and Stent are topics that were prescribed by doctor to all of the 95 patients, that undergone surgery (PCI: angioplasty and stent placement). In addition to the main information on the diseases and intervention totally Majority of topics offered to the patients in this study were about surgery (27.5%), treatment (25%), General topics related to CAD and other information on (24.6%). The lowest percentage of topics prescribed for patients was about diagnosis techniques (8.9%), and after that about medicines (14%).

6. Drivers and barriers

Influencing factors were categorized into two groups: drivers and barriers. Some of the factors can act dual functionally in other word their presence helps the progress of process and their absence cut down and create difficulty for service. In such cases border line may be drown case vise.

6.1 Drivers

6.1.1 Patients' preference and demand for Information

6.1.2 Physician's interest and belief on providing IPs to patients

6.1.3 Number of Information specialist who are interested in Filling information prescriptions

6.1.4 Availability of more than 80% of demanded information

6.2 Barriers

6.2.1. Time: Time is the most critical component of information Therapy service . Ideally there should not be time gap between oral information that a physician gives to a patient and the information prescription which is Filled for patient. In the most preferred situation IP would better to be given to patient at the 10-15 minute visit time. IP also can be given along with the medications and Rx.

6.2.2. Integrated health information system (HIS): In an integrated HIS all the components of databases are coded, for example: ICD10 is used for coding diseases, NDC for drug, CPT for diagnostic tests and NLM for information. Coding enables the flow and circulation of information easy, fast and secure thought the system. In this project lack of such integrated system was crucial.

6.2.3 Confidence: confidence between health providers and patient is a two edge factor either driver or barrier for Ix and IPs.

6.2.4 Place: An identified place with at least 2 computer systems , internet connection, printer (color and or back and with) to receive, prepare and deliver prescriptions on time

6.2.5 ICT applications: Low speed internet connection is a critical barrier for successful Ix and IP services.

6.2.6 Mobile Technology: Mobile computer and mobile phone facilitate availability and accessibility of information. A mobile phone with printer can create shift in IPs service in ward round. Patient in developing countries use mobile phone more than web and they demand for mobile phone information delivery more than web or email delivery (Vishwa M., Gavgan V.Z, 2009).

6.2.7 Database: Database of patient information is critical driver for Ix and IP services. Without having reliable information accessible, IP services will be time consuming process.

6.2.8 Patients's portal: Patient portal makes information available either from outside sources or from patient interactions.

6.2.9 Organizational support: Without organizational support , coordination and management it is impossible to practice Ix and IP in countries with centralized government and health system. We had limitation to take part in ward round or have access to patients' data because clinical librarianship concept does not practice formally in Iran.

6.2.10 Multimedia format: Availability of information in multimedia format is effective and efficient tool in understanding, learning and practicing prescribed information.

6.2.11 Literacy : Rural population are almost illiterate and it can be considered barrier if information supposed to be given in print format. Having information stored in different formats like audio and or audiovisual files can be used/offered in along with IP for better understanding.

6.2.12 Budget: Allocating money is also helpful in different aspects. It can be used in Critical situation that IPs team may face in providing and offering the service more effectively.

6.2.13 Confidentiality: Confidentiality is vital at least in patients-doctor relationship. Patient should be given guarantee that their health, mental and physical data is kept secure and will be used only for better health care. In some cases patients were worried about why should they are asking for specific questions and why should they are offered with specific information.

6.2.14 Communication style: In hospital setting clinicians give information about diseases and medications to patients orally. In conscious assent also it is usual to briefly explain the probable side effects, non effect and harms of intervention especially for surgery. But it is believed that the communication style, stress and pressure on words and procedures may effect in preference of patients (Nabhan A ,2011). Written information is documented and does not stress on type of intervention directly or indirectly.

7. Conclusion

The main Objective of this project was provision of IPs for patients with cardiovascular problems. The project successfully was conducted and the process of execution illustrated using flowchart. The other objective of study was finding drivers and barriers for IPs in Iran as a sample of developing country with lack of required facilities like electronic health record (EHR) and patient information services. The study found that despite of patients' preference and interest in receiving IPs, there are limitations for fulfillment of IPs in developing countries like Iran. Access to the Internet, electronic and integrated health records, patient information portals, availability of computer for individuals, health and computer literacy, are inconsistent throughout country. Therefore, it is essential to adopt both traditional paper based system and Information technology along with emerging IT based tools to ensure sustainability of IPs. The most significant barrier for Ix and IP service we faced in this project was cultural change and attitude of stakeholders including physicians, health providers and health consumers. Although physicians and nurses accept the theory of Ix and IP service and believe that patient has right to information and right information at right time to be made available for them. In practice they feel uncomfortable with it. Some of the health providers think that giving information to patients may create more and unnecessary jobs for health providers. Next to this issues the technical problems can be categorized in three including: 1) Time 2) Health information Technology and system 3) Training. Physicians time to accomplish IPs affected by many interconnected factors. One of the factors can be availability ICT and HIS. The last, HIS, is itself a big issue. Without HIS and patient information database/system it is very difficult for physicians to prescribe information even if they are appetite to empower their patients and get their feedbacks for shared decision making. Therefore; it can be said that at time, the biggest barrier to accomplish IPs in non wired and non-English language countries like Iran is lack of Patient Information system in vernacular languages like Persian. At least a patient information database is a significant factor to store, retrieve and personalize patient information in vernacular language at the moment of care. To overcome the time barrier on the side of physicians it is essential to consider the IPs as a essential component of physicians-patient communication in any visit .Physicians and residents need to be trained in prescription of information to their patients and other allied health providers like nurses also need to be trained to recognize the importance of IP s and its differences with the longstanding patient education in their profession. This study suggests that, to practice Ix and IPs successfully it is essential to create a framework in healthcare system in which every stakeholder and every particle of system including physician, nurse, informationist, social workers and patient look at health care promotion as a continual quality improvement goal. Patient care and information prescription need to be accepted as a best practice to empower patient. Protocols and guideline to be developed and made available for health providers and other stakeholders to enable them practiced Ix and IPs based of their own specific environment according to the facilities, barriers, cultural and ideological issues.

8. References

Kemper, D.W. & Mettler, M. (2002a). Information Therapy prescribing the right information to the right person at the right time. *Managed Care Quarterly*, 10(4).

Gavgani V.Z. (2011). Information Therapy (Ix) and patients' preference. IGI Publishing Group. *International Journal of Computational Models and Algorithms in Medicine (IJCMAM)*;2(2):42-50.

Gavgani V.Z. (2010-2011). An investigation to find out attitude of clinical faculty members about prescription of information patients therapy ; Unpublished research Project approved by Tabriz University of medical sciences-research deputy department. Code of ethics committee 5/4/8685.

Asr Iran (2011).The latest situation of Internet Speed in Iran and Other countries . *Asr Iran Newsletter20th* othdibehesht , news code 165184. Retrieved from < http://www.asriran.com/fa/news/165184. >

A subject vise Hadith Databank (2011) Retrieve from < http://www.aviny.com/hadis-mozooee/ejtemai/salamati.aspx>

Tebyan (2011). Nutriotin and health in Quran and hadith. Retrieved from < http://www.tebyan.net/index.aspx?pid=65874>

Nabhan A. (2011). Impact of reporting the number treated needlessly on perceived effectiveness and decision to adopt an intervention. 19th Cochrane Colloquium; Internation Conference on Patient Safety. 19-22 October 2011. Madrid . Retrieved from <http://colloquium.cochrane.org/abstracts/a2o1-impact-reporting-number-treated-needlessly-perceived-effectiveness-and-decision-adopt>

Gavgani, V.Z. (2009). "Role of medical Librarians in information Therapy (Ix): study of problems and prospects in India and Iran". PhD.Thesis submitted to Osmania University, Hyderabad - India.

Gavgani V.Z. (2011). Role of librarians in information therapy (Ix): a comparative study of two developing countries. *Aslib Proceedings: New Information Perspectives* Vol. 63 (6): 603-617. DOI 10.1108/00012531111187252 Retrieved from < http://www.emeraldinsight.com/journals.htm?issn=0001-253x&volume=63&issue=6&articleid=17004119&show=abstrac >

Gavgani VZ (2011). 2nd conference of Information Therapy to put patient at first Prescription of Information for patient with Coronary Artery Disease. 9th October Mumbai-India. Retrieved from < http://patientpower.in/ >

Kemper D.W. , Metler M.(2002b). Information Therapy:prescribed information as a reimbursable medical service, Boise, Healthwise.

Vishwa M, Gavgani V.Z. (2009) "Informing Clients Through ICT" . Issues in Informing Science and Information Technology, 6 :585-592. Retrieved from <http://iisit.org/Vol6/IISITv6p585-593Mohan622.pdf>

7

Changing Attitudes in Obstetrics and Gynecology – How Evidence Based Medicine is Changing Our Practice?

Hesham Al-Inany and Amr Wahba
Cairo University Hospital,
Egypt

1. Introduction

Evidence-based medicine (EBM) is the process of systematically reviewing, appraising and using clinical research findings to aid the delivery of optimum clinical care to patients (Rosenberg and Donald, 1995). It is considered a new trend in both teaching medicine and supporting the clinical decisive process, answering the clinical questions. The basis of the evidence-based medicine comprises of analysing and interpreting current and reliable medical publications concerning certain subject (Laudański and Pierzyński., 2000).

Evidence-based practice is "a process of care that takes the patient and his or her preferences and actions, the clinical setting including the resources available, and current and applicable scientific evidence, and knits the three together using the clinical expertise and training of the health-care providers." (Haynes *et al.*, 2002).

Thus, EBP as illustrated in Figure (1) is the integration of *clinical expertise, patient values*, and the *best research evidence* into the decision making process for patient care. Clinical expertise refers to the clinician's cumulated experience, education and clinical skills. The patient brings to the encounter his or her own personal and unique concerns, expectations, and values. The best evidence is usually found in clinically relevant research that has been conducted using sound methodology (Sackett *et al.*, 2000).

Despite its ancient origins, evidence based medicine remains a relatively young discipline whose positive impacts are just beginning to be validated, and it will continue to evolve (Bennett *et al.*, 1987; Shin *et al.*, 1993).

The aim of this chapter is to explore different aspects of evidence based medicine including background on its development, motives towards changing our attitudes in practice and how can evidence be extracted. The chapter will also highlight the major role of evidence based medicine in changing attitudes towards evidence based practice which ensures safety and efficiency of the health service provided, in the field of obstetrics and gynecology; a domain that has greatly participated in the establishment of evidence based medicine and evidence based practice. Many examples on how evidence based medicine has changed attitudes in practice will be displayed to demonstrate and emphasize this role.

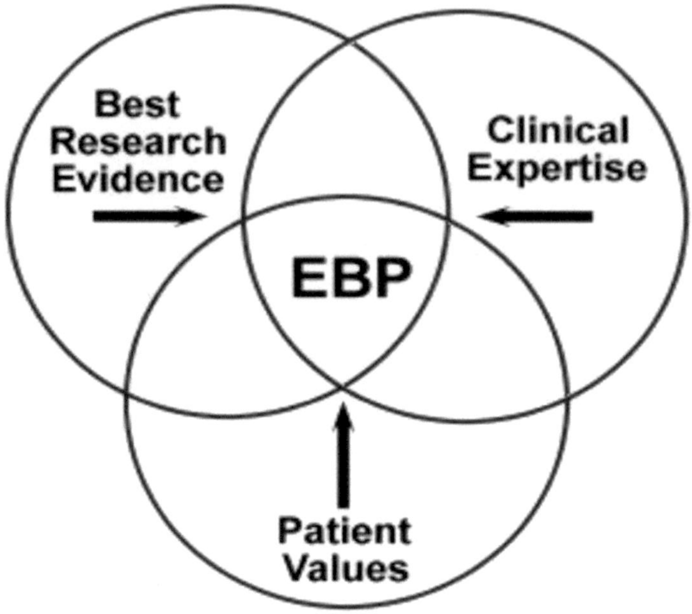

Fig. 1. Evidence Based Practice (EBP)

2. Why changing attitudes in practice

Although clinical research is consistently producing new findings that may contribute to effective and efficient patient care, the findings of such research will not change population outcomes unless health services and health care professionals adopt them in practice (Grimshaw *et al.*, 2001).

However, the enormous volume of information that is published in an ever-increasing number of available medical journals constitute a major obstacle and a real challenge to obtaining reliable evidence for clinical practice from research. Over half a million papers on gynecology, infertility, pregnancy and obstetrics are published each year. To sift through these MEDLINE records, let alone the full papers that may be relevant, to identify those which should form the basis of clinical practice is an overwhelming and nearly impossible task. How, then, can busy clinicians have easy access to, and identify, the most appropriate information on which to base their clinical decisions? (Dodd and Crowther, 2006).

The contribution of evidence-based medicine to improved patient outcomes in general practice is incontestable. Evidence based practice promotes practices that have better outcomes and are scientifically proven to be effective. It aims to eliminate unsound or risky practices, thus improving quality of care, providing best service to the patient and promoting patient safety.

Actually, evidence based practice is one step toward making sure that each patient gets the best service possible. Furthermore, it helps physicians to keep knowledge up to date and supplements clinical judgment; very vital benefit especially in the light of the rapidly growing literature and medical advances.

3. Evidence based and experience oriented practice

Clinical medicine is currently in transition from experience-oriented practice to an evidence-based one which requires the best available evidence that answers our clinical questions for better safety and efficacy. However, there is a balance, and even tension, between evidence and clinical expertise:

"Without clinical expertise, practice risks becoming tyrannized by external evidence, for even excellent external evidence may be inapplicable to or inappropriate for an individual patient. Without current best external evidence, practice risks becoming rapidly out of date, to the detriment of patients." Good doctors use both individual clinical expertise and the best available external evidence, and neither alone is enough (Sackett et al., 1996).

Evidence based medicine helps clinicians to integrate the best external clinical evidence from systematic research with individual clinical expertise to make effective decisions about patient treatment and care.

Best available external clinical evidence means clinically relevant research, often from the basic sciences of medicine, but especially from patient centred clinical research into the accuracy and precision of diagnostic tests, the power of prognostic markers, and the efficacy and safety of therapeutic, rehabilitative, and preventive regimens.

External clinical evidence can inform, but can never replace, individual clinical expertise, and it is this expertise that decides whether the external evidence applies to the individual patient at all and, if so, how it should be integrated into a clinical decision (Sackett *et al.*, 1996).

4. How can evidence be extracted?

The best evidence is usually found in clinically relevant research that has been conducted using sound methodology (Sackett *et al.*, 2000). EBM is not restricted to randomized trials and meta-analyses. Actually, it involves tracking down the best external evidence with which to answer our clinical questions.

Thus, to find out about the accuracy of a *diagnostic test*, we need to find proper cross-sectional studies of patients clinically suspected of harboring the relevant disorder, not a randomized trial while for a question about *prognosis*, we need proper follow-up studies (i.e. prospective cohort studies) of patients assembled at a uniform, early point in the clinical course of their disease. And, sometimes, the evidence we need will come from the basic sciences, such as genetics or immunology.

It is when asking questions about *therapy* that we should try to avoid the non-experimental approaches, because these routinely lead to false-positive conclusions about efficacy. Because the randomized trial, and especially the systematic review of several randomized trials, is so much more likely to inform us and so much less likely to mislead us, it has become the "**gold standard**" for judging whether a treatment does more good than harm (Sackett et al., 1996).

5. Development of evidence based practice in obstetrics

Although the term 'evidence-based medicine' was first used by Gordon Guyatt of McMaster University, Canada, in 1990, (Guyatt and Rennie, 2002) the development of evidence-based practice in obstetrics began in the early 1970s. Archie Cochrane, in his now well-known writings (Cochrane, 1972), awarded the 'wooden spoon' to obstetricians for having made the poorest use of randomized controlled trials, and having widely incorporated changes into clinical practice without appropriate evaluation(Cochrane, 1972).

Such observation inspired Iain Chalmers in 1974 to start the enormous task of collecting all randomized controlled trials related to the field of perinatal medicine. More than 3000 trials conducted between 1940 and 1984 were identified. This collection was first published in 1985 as the Oxford Database of Perinatal Trials (ODPT) (Chlamers *et al.*, 1986). In 1989, the first comprehensive synthesis of evidence for pregnancy care, entitled "Effective Care in Pregnancy and Childbirth" (ECPC), was published; it included systematic reviews of the identified randomized trials (Enkin *et al.*, 1989).

This two-volume book was condensed into the paperback "A Guide to Effective Care in Pregnancy and Childbirth (GECPC)" summarizing the available evidence on the effects of pregnancy care, and categorizing care practices into those with evidence of known benefit, those of uncertain benefit, and those of known harm (Enkin *et al.*, 1989). All of these early pregnancy and childbirth initiatives were important forerunners to the Cochrane Collaboration (The Cochrane Library, 2005).

6. Examples for how evidence based medicine changed practices in obstetrics and gynecology

We will be displaying in the coming section many practical examples elaborating the great noticeable role of evidence based medicine in shifting the practices in obstetrics and gynecology towards better safety and higher efficacy and in eliminating risky unsafe practices. Evidence based medicine has changed attitudes towards interventions, therapeutics and diagnostics.

6.1 Changing attitudes towards interventions (evidence based interventions)

What matters in health care is identifying and using interventions that have been shown by strong research evidence to achieve the best outcomes within available resources for everyone (Fletcher and Lancet, 1999). Examples for such interventions will be discussed.

6.1.1 The term breech trial

Among most issues in the field of obstetrics that have been very controversial is the breech delivery. Approximately 4% of all infants are in breech presentation. Delivery in this position is more difficult, with increased risk of complications to the fetus such as umbilical cord prolapse, hypoxia, and fetal injury.

Despite increased risks, breech deliveries are usually accomplished without complications and without the need for 'expert assistance' from an experienced, trained clinician or midwife. However, in the event that expert assistance is needed but not obtained, permanent damage can occur during breech births because of the lack of appropriate and well-timed actions by the birth attendant.

Historically, vaginal breech deliveries were considered the norm until 1959, when routine cesarean delivery was shown to reduce perinatal mortality and morbidity (Wright, 1959).

While there was a general belief that planned cesarean delivery was better than planned vaginal delivery for breech deliveries, evidence was inconclusive because most studies were observational, two small RCTs showed no difference, and evidence suggested that improved neonatal outcomes might occur at the expense of poorer maternal outcomes.

The Term Breech trial, a multi-center trial across 121 centers in 26 countries randomizing 2088 women to 'planned cesarean delivery' or 'planned vaginal' deliveries (1997 - 2000). The trial found during interim analyses that cesarean delivery was associated with a reduced risk of perinatal morbidity and mortality. The term breech trial had an immediate **dramatic impact** on the management of term breech deliveries with policies changed in accordance with the trials findings. Rapid change in clinical practice occurred in many locations, although not universally, as some desired more evidence and others were reticent to accept the trials results as conclusive (Hannah *et al.*, 2000).

Several comparison studies showed alteration of clinical practice via examining rates of vaginal breech delivery versus cesarean delivery in various countries (e.g., New Zealand, Australia) (Kaushik and Gudgeon, 2003).

6.1.2 Examples of other obstetrical interventions

There was widespread variation in clinical practice in areas such as the role of external cephalic version (ECV) for breech presentation (effective in reducing the need for caesarean delivery), the use of prophylactic antibiotics at caesarean delivery (effective in reducing maternal puerperal sepsis), the use of antenatal corticosteroids for fetal lung maturation (effective in reducing the risk of neonatal respiratory disease and mortality in infants born preterm), the use of vacuum-assisted vaginal births (effective in reducing maternal vaginal and perineal trauma), and selective versus routine use of episiotomy (effective in reducing maternal perineal trauma).

The systematic reviews first published in Effective Care in Pregnancy and Childbirth (ECPC) and The Oxford Database of Perinatal Trials (ODPT), and by the Cochrane Collaboration Pregnancy and Childbirth review group, summarized the best available evidence at the time, indicating benefit for all of these interventions. For some of these interventions, clinical practice has indeed changed.

Prenatal corticosteroids are now widely prescribed for women at risk of preterm birth, with 82% of mothers of infants born at less than 34 weeks' gestation admitted to the neonatal intensive care unit in Australia, having been administered corticosteroids prior to birth (Donoghue *et al.*, 2002). The uptake of ECV for breech presentation at term has been less successful, with only 67% of obstetricians surveyed in Australia and New Zealand offering ECV (Phipps *et al.*, 2003).

6.1.3 The obstetrical outcomes after conservative treatment of intraepithelial neoplasia or early invasive lesions

With the establishment of effective screening programmes for cancer cervix, women are more commonly diagnosed early with preinvasive lesions and microinvasive cervical cancers which make younger women with such lesions candidate for conservative treatment for the sake of preservation of the potential for childbearing.

However, proper counseling of those young women on the effect of such conservative treatment on the obstetrical outcome has been problematic and inadequate till the emergence of an important **meta-analysis** performed by Kyrgiou *et al* in 2006 in which the authors have investigated the obstetric outcomes in women who underwent excisional procedures in the cervix (Kyrgiou *et al.*, 2006).

In this meta-anlaysis, a total of 27 studies were included. The authors exhibited that cold knife cervical conisation was significantly associated with preterm delivery, low birth weight and cesarean delivery; similarly Large Loop Excision of the Transformation Zone (LLETZ) was associated with preterm delivery, low birth weight and premature rupture of the membranes. Similar but marginally non-significant adverse effects were recorded for laser conisation. But the investigators did not detect significantly increased risks for obstetric outcomes after laser ablation.

It was concluded that all the excisional procedures used to treat cervical intraepithelial neoplasia present similar pregnancy-related morbidity without apparent neonatal morbidity. This study changed the future attitude of gynecologists towards women with abnormal cervical lesions and alerted the physicians to be more cautious for future treatment options. This study also provided clinicians with evidence base to counsel women appropriately (Kyrgiou *et al.*, 2006).

6.1.4 Preimplantation genetic screening for aneuploidies in IVF/ICSI

Despite the great advances that have taken place in the field of in vitro fertilization (IVF) since its introduction in 1978 with the achievement of considerable success rates in almost all causes of infertility, still many women fail to become pregnant in spite of repeated transfers of apparently morphologically normal embryos.

Among the highly accused causes for this repeated failure is the inherent abnormal chromosomal make-up of the embryos (i.e. embryonic aneuploidy) (Wilton, 2002). Other causes responsible for the pregnancy failure are the poor endometrial receptivity and the inefficiency of the embryo transfer techniques (Mansour and Aboulghar, 2002).

Many of the chromosome abnormalities observed in human embryos will cause the embryos to die early in development, sometimes even before implantation, or before term pregnancy can be reached.

Patient populations with certain characteristics (e.g. advanced maternal age, recurrent implantation failure , repeated miscarriages, patients undergoing testicular sperm extraction (TESE) and intracytoplasmic sperm injection (ICSI) have been considered at higher risk of producing aneuploid embryos (Kahraman *et al.*, 2004; Munne *et al.*, 2004; Gianaroli *et al.*, 2005) which would die around the time of implantation and therefore result in no established pregnancy (Munne *et al.*, 2003; Caglar *et al.*, 2005).

In recent years, these observations of significant incidences of aneuploidy in early human embryos has led to the expansion of preimplantation genetic diagnosis techniques for aneuploidies (PGD-AS) to patients who are considered to have a poor prognosis of reaching a full-term pregnancy (Sermon *et al.*, 2005).

Embryo morphology alone cannot be used to predict euploidy since many good quality embryos have been found to be aneuploid (Delhanty *et al.*, 1997; Harper *et al.*, 1995; Magli *et al.*, 2001), thus genetic diagnosis is required to detect aneuploid embryos.

Two main techniques namely; fluorescent in situ hybridization (FISH) for multiple chromosomes and polymerase chain reaction (PCR), are used to document a high frequency of chromosomal errors and aneuploidy in human preimplantation embryos. These techniques enable the selection of chromosomally normal embryos that are more likely to implant.

PGD-AS is commonly also known as preimplantation genetic screening (PGS), with both terms used interchangeably. PGS needs to be differentiated from preimplantation genetic diagnosis (PGD). While the technology used in both techniques is almost identical, PGS and PGD differ mainly in their indications. PGD aims to prevent the birth of affected children in couples with a high risk of transmitting specific genetic disorders, whether numerical or structural in nature. PGS, on the other hand, aims to improve pregnancy rates in infertile couples undergoing IVF/ICSI treatment, and who do not have any chromosomal aberrations.

PGS allows the detection of aneuploidy before the step of embryo transfer. Aneuploid embryos could be screened out and only euploid ones transferred, thus theoretically increasing the chance of pregnancy and reducing the chance of miscarriage.

A recent systematic review and meta-analysis by **Abou-Setta *et al.***, in 2011 aimed to evaluate whether PGS can improve the clinical outcomes of IVF/ICSI compared with no intervention. There was no significant difference in live birth rates following PGS compared with no PGS (R.R = 0.79, 95% CI: 0.54 to 1.15; p = 0.22; I^2 = 65.74%, 95% uCI: 10.51% to 86.89%) (Figure 2). As well, there was no significant difference in clinical pregnancy rate following PGS compared with no PGS (R.R = 0.89, 95% CI: 0.67 to 1.17; p = 0.40; I^2 = 62.00%, 95% uCI: 1.70% to 76.66%) (Figure 3).

	PGS		Control			Risk Ratio
Study or Subgroup	Events	Total	Events	Total	Weight	M-H, Random, 95% CI
Blockeel 2008	15	95	25	105	18.9%	0.66 [0.37, 1.18]
Hardarson 2008	3	56	10	53	7.4%	0.28 [0.08, 0.98]
Mastenbroek 2007	22	206	36	202	21.4%	0.60 [0.37, 0.98]
Schoolcraft 2009	25	32	20	30	27.3%	1.17 [0.86, 1.60]
Staessen 2008	37	120	37	120	25.1%	1.00 [0.68, 1.46]
Total (95% CI)		**509**		**510**	**100.0%**	**0.79 [0.54, 1.15]**
Total events	102		128			

Heterogeneity: $Tau^2 = 0.11$; $Chi^2 = 11.68$, df = 4 (P = 0.02); $I^2 = 66\%$
Test for overall effect: Z = 1.22 (P = 0.22)

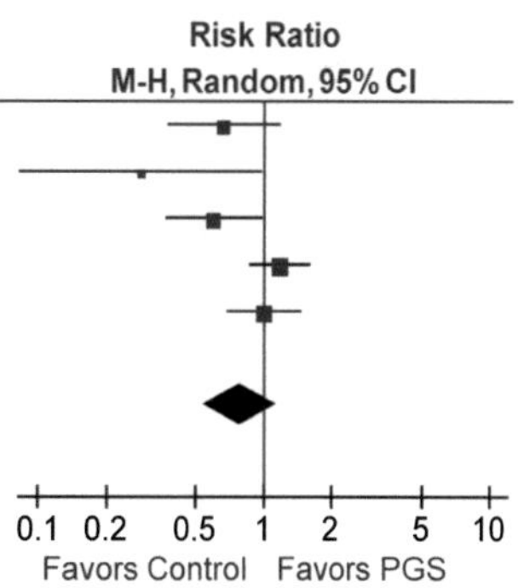

Fig. 2. Forest plot of comparison: PGS vs Control Live birth rate

The results of this systematic review showed that until today, there was no enough evidence in the literature to give a conclusive decision on the value of PGS for patients undergoing IVF/ICSI. Currently with the evidence at hand, PGS seems to have no impact on improving live birth rate (Figure 2) and the clinical pregnancy rate (Figure 3) in patients undergoing IVF/ICSI. In fact, many of the trials were not completed and were stopped early because of the ineffectiveness of the intervention **(Abou-setta *et al.*, 2011).**

	PGS		Control			Risk Ratio
Study or Subgroup	Events	Total	Events	Total	Weight	M-H, Random, 95% CI
Blockeel 2008	18	95	28	105	13.0%	0.71 [0.42, 1.20]
Hardarson 2008	5	56	13	53	6.2%	0.36 [0.14, 0.95]
Mastenbroek 2007	34	206	46	202	16.1%	0.72 [0.49, 1.08]
Schoolcraft 2009	25	32	20	30	18.6%	1.17 [0.86, 1.60]
Scott 2010	12	13	9	15	15.0%	1.54 [0.99, 2.39]
Staessen 2004	25	200	29	200	13.6%	0.86 [0.52, 1.42]
Staessen 2008	38	120	46	120	17.6%	0.83 [0.58, 1.17]
Total (95% CI)		**722**		**725**	**100.0%**	**0.89 [0.67, 1.17]**
Total events	157		191			

Heterogeneity: $Tau^2 = 0.08$; $Chi^2 = 15.93$, df = 6 (P = 0.01); $I^2 = 62\%$

Test for overall effect: Z = 0.84 (P = 0.40)

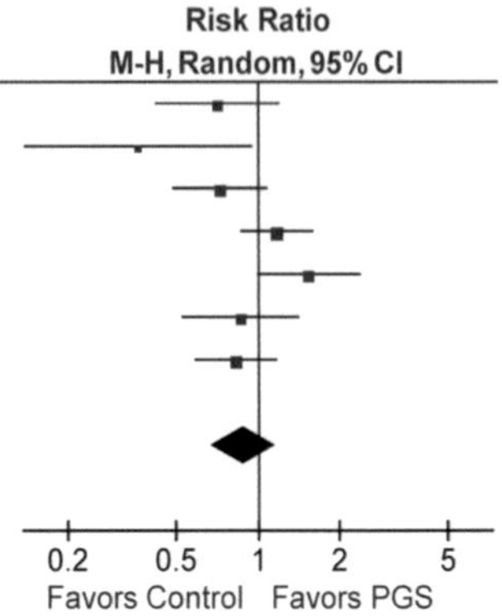

Fig. 3. Forest plot of comparison: PGS Vs Control Clinical pregnancy rate

6.2 Changing attitudes towards therapeutics (evidence based therapeutics)

The advances in therapeutics are tremendous with many novel drugs and therapies manufactured and developed every day with the emergence of new strategies and mechanisms of actions making the selection of the best effective therapy a difficult and challenging task. Evaluation of the superiority of a particular therapy based on a single trial is inadequate and deficient. Hence, for evaluation to be better and adequate, it should be served by a comprehensive and systematic review of all existing data sets. We will display examples for some therapeutics that have been evaluated in an evidence based approach, resulting in changing attitudes towards their use.

6.2.1 Hormone Replacement Therapy: WHI study

Hormone replacement therapy, (HRT) involves the replacement of the depleted hormone levels in menopausal women by the administration of synthetic estrogen with or without progestogen with the aim to alleviate symptoms of menopause.

Despite the potential health benefits that were expected from the use of HRT, many risks and complications have been associated with its use. Although observational studies suggested protective effects on heart disease (Stampfer *et al.*, 1991), osteoporosis (Lindsay *et al.*, 1976), and even Alzheimer's disease (Henderson *et al.*, 1994), recent clinical trials have questioned some of these benefits. Till now, the debate regarding the risk-benefit ratio of hormone replacement therapy has not been completely resolved.

However, in July 2002, the Women's Health Initiative (WHI), - a large, multicentric clinical trial by the National Heart, Lung and Blood Institute (NHLBI) and other units of National Institute of Health (NIH) – reported that hormone replacement therapy actually posed more health risks than benefits (Rossouw *et al.*, 2002).

This was **the turning point** in HRT, as the number of health hazards attributed to HRT grew, practitioners discontinued routine prescriptions for this once a time very popular and rampant treatment modality and HRT use substantially decreased in the general population (Dorval *et al.*, 2007, Hersh *et al.*, 2004, Majumdar *et al.*, 2004).

The results of this study provide the best evidence available at present on HRT for prevention of heart disease, and indicate that combined HRT is not indicated for this purpose in the studied population, thus contradicting the reported beneficial effects of HRT on coronary heart disease (CHD) in previous observational studies (Rossouw *et al.*, 2002).

6.2.2 Inudction of ovulation in patients with polycystic ovary syndrome

Polycystic ovary syndrome has an estimated prevalence of 4-8 % in reproductive-aged women (Knochenhauer *et al.*, 1998; Asuncion *et al.*, 2000). It is the most common cause of oligoanovulatory infertility (Hull, 1987). Ovulation in these cases has been suggested to be induced by the use of clomiphene citrate or insulin sensitizer or combination of both.

Metformin as an insulin sensitizer improves peripheral insulin sensitivity by decreasing glucose production by the liver and increasing the sensitivity of target tissues to insulin. Metformin was also found to reduce levels of androgens in both lean and obese women, leading to increased rates of spontaneous ovulation (Batukan *et al.*, 2001; Haas *et al.*, 2003; Essah *et al.*, 2006).

It has been demonstrated by a number of studies that up to 40 % of anovulatory women with polycystic ovary syndrome will ovulate, and many will achieve pregnancy with metformin alone (Diamanti-Kandarakis *et al.*, 1998; Neveu *et al.*, 2007).

Despite the postulated effectiveness of metformin in induction of ovulation in cases with polycystic ovary syndrome, randomised controlled trials conducted by Moll et al., 2006 and Legro et al., 2007 didn't support these expectations.

Moll *et al.*, 2006 performed a randomised double blind clinical trial to compare the effect of clomiphene citrate plus metformin and clomiphene citrate plus placebo on induction of ovulation in women with newly diagnosed polycystic ovary syndrome. The authors recruited 228 women with polycystic ovary syndrome, of those, 111 women were allocated to clomiphene citrate plus metformin (metformin group) and 114 women were allocated to clomiphene citrate plus placebo (placebo group).

The results of the study showed that the ovulation rate in the metformin group was 64% compared with 72% in the placebo group, a non-significant difference (risk difference − 8%, 95% confidence interval − 20% to 4%). Hence, the authors concluded that metformin is not an effective addition to clomiphene citrate as the primary method of inducing ovulation in women with polycystic ovary syndrome.

The above conclusion was also emphasized by another study performed by Legro *et al.* in 2007 who conducted a randomized prospective study involving 626 infertile women with polycystic ovary syndrome. In this study, the authors found live-birth rates with clomiphene citrate alone were higher (22.5 %) than with metformin alone (7.2 %) (Legro *et al.*, 2007).

6.2.3 Metformin in prevention of ovarian hyperstimulation syndrome

Ovarian hyperstimulation syndrome (OHSS) is considered to be the most serious complication of superovulation in IVF-embryo transfer. The syndrome can vary in presentation from mild to severe life threatening disease. Severe manifestations of OHSS may include massive fluid shifts, hemoconcentration or renal and liver dysfunction. The syndrome may be ultimately complicated by thromboembolic events and adult respiratory distress syndrome (Rizk and Aboulghar, 1999).

Several strategies have been suggested to prevent such life threatening complication of ovulation induction. Among the suggested strategies is the administration of metformin. A **meta-analysis** has indicated that the administration of metformin significantly prevents OHSS development in patients with polycystic ovary syndrome, a high risk group (Costello *et al.*, 2006).

The mechanism of action of metformin is not completely clear, but both reduction of ovarian reserve, as demonstrated by the reduction of anti-Müllerian hormone (AMH) values (Piltonen *et al.*, 2005), and a reduced insulin dependent VEGF production (Tang *et al.*, 2006), have been suggested.

6.2.4 Changing attitudes in ovarian stimulation towards patient's safety

Gonadotropin-releasing hormone agonists (GnRHa) were introduced in ovarian stimulation for IVF to suppress the premature surge of luteinizing hormone (LH).

Various protocols have been suggested for controlled ovarian hyperstimulation in assisted reproduction, however, the long agonist protocol have been the standard protocol because of the associated increase in pregnancy rates.

In this long agonist protocol, GnRHa is started either in the mid-luteal phase or in the early follicular phase of the preceding cycle and continued until pituitary desensitization has been achieved; usually after 2–3 weeks, at which point gonadotropin administration will be started (Al-Inany and Aboulghar, 2003).

However, despite the increased pregnancy rates, the use of the GnRHa long protocols has been concurrently associated with an increase in the incidence of ovarian hyperstimulation syndrome (Rizk and Smitz, 1992).

The fear from such serious and potentially life threatening complications has motivated researchers to study other alternative protocols that would achieve better safety with at least equivalent results, thus improving the outcome of IVF. Gonadotropin-releasing hormone antagonists have emerged as an alternative treatment for preventing premature LH surges during controlled ovarian hyperstimulation (Al-Inany *et al.*, 2011).

GnRH agonist and antagonist exert their effects through different mechanisms of action. GnRH agonists act by downregulation of pituitary GnRH receptors and desensitization of the gonadotropic cells, while GnRH antagonists act by directly and rapidly inhibiting gonadotropin release within several hours through competitive binding to pituitary GnRH receptors. This mechanism of action is dependent on the equilibrium between endogenous GnRH and the applied antagonist and is highly dose dependent in contrast to the agonists (Felberbaum *et al.*, 1995).

The competitive blockade of the receptors by GnRH antagonists results in immediate arrest of gonadotropin secretion; therefore, they can be given after starting gonadotropin administration. This will lead to dramatic reduction in the duration of treatment cycle as well as avoiding flare up and estrogen deprivation symptoms associated with GnRHa-induced downregulation.

Cochrane reviews comparing GnRH antagonist to the more widely used long GnRH agonist protocols were published successively, with the first review published in 2001 (Al-Inany and Aboulghar, 2001), that was later updated in 2006 (Al-Inany *et al.*, 2006) and recently updated again in 2011 (Al-Inany *et al.*, 2011). The last updated review focused on patient-oriented value mainly safety and ongoing pregnancy/live birth rate.

The earlier two versions of that review showed lower efficacy for GnRH antagonists while the most recent one showed lower pregnancy in antagonist but did not reach statistically significant level.

According to the most recent review, nine trials reported live birth rates in 1515 women. There was no significant difference in live birth rates following GnRH antagonist compared with GnRH agonist (OR = 0.86, 95% CI = 0.69 to 1.08; p = 0.20; I^2 = 0.00%, 95% CI = 0.00% to 31.62%) (Figure 3).

However, more importantly, there were a statistically highly significant lower incidence of OHSS in the GnRH antagonist group (Twenty-nine randomized controlled trials reported ovarian hyperstimulation rates in 5417 women, R.D = -0.03, 95% CI = -0.05 to -0.02; $p < 0.00001$; I2 = 67,68%, 95% CI = 52.50% to 78.02%) (See Figure 4).

Thus, there was a significant difference favouring GnRH antagonist compared with GnRH agonist. The incidence was reduced by 50% in antagonist group (1.91 vs 3.74%). The corresponding number needed to harm was 25 (95% CI: 19–36) with an absolute risk reduction of 4% (95% CI: 2.79–5.13).

This means that for every 25 women undergoing downregulation by agonist, one more case of severe OHSS may be expected. In addition, the cancellation rate owing to high risk to develop OHSS was significantly higher in GnRHa group. This means that the difference would be highly significant if cancellation was not done (Al-Inany *et al.*, 2011).

6.2.5 For intrauterine insemination (IUI) timing: Which is the best; human chorionic gonadotropin administration or monitoring of LH surge?

Kosmas *et al.*, 2007 conducted a systematic review and meta-anlaysis to find out whether the timing of intrauterine insemination by the administration of hCG achieves better results than the monitoring of LH surge.

Seven studies with 2,623 patients were involved in this meta-analysis, in which 1,461 patients received hCG, and 1,162 had LH surge detection. When all studies were combined, patients who received hCG before IUI demonstrated lower clinical-pregnancy rates than did women who had IUI after spontaneous ovulation (odds ratio, 0.74; 95% confidence interval, 0.57–0.961).

In subgroup analysis of studies that considered ovulatory dysfunction to be the infertility reason, the results favored women who received hCG. In contrast, across studies that reported male factor as the infertility reason, as well as across studies including women with unexplained infertility, results appeared to favor the LH surge detection approach. However, none of those subgroup analyses reached statistical significance (Kosmas *et al.*, 2007).

Study or Subgroup	GnRH antagonist Events	Total	GnRH agonist Events	Total	Weight	Odds Ratio M-H, Fixed, 95% CI
1.1.1 All women						
Albano 2000	34	198	19	95	13.5%	0.83 [0.44, 1.55]
Barmat 2005	13	40	17	40	7.3%	0.65 [0.26, 1.62]
Heijnen 2007	70	205	78	199	33.0%	0.80 [0.54, 1.21]
Hurine 2006	17	91	17	91	8.8%	1.00 [0.47, 2.11]
Kim 2009	13	54	8	28	5.1%	0.79 [0.28, 2.22]
Kurzawa 2008	14	37	18	37	7.1%	0.64 [0.25, 1.62]
Lin 2006	22	60	21	60	8.4%	1.08 [0.51, 2.27]
Marci 2005	4	30	0	30	0.3%	10.36 [0.53, 201.45]
Ye 2009	35	109	39	111	16.6%	0.87 [0.50, 1.53]
Subtotal (95% CI)		**824**		**691**	**100.0%**	**0.86 [0.69, 1.08]**
Total events	222		217			
Heterogeneity: $Chi^2 = 4.09$, df = 8 (P = 0.85); $I^2 = 0\%$						
Test for overall effect: Z = 1.27 (P = 0.20)						
1.1.2 Minimal stimulation IVF only						
Heijnen 2007	75	205	81	199	79.7%	0.84 [0.56, 1.25]
Lin 2006	22	60	21	60	20.3%	1.08 [0.51, 2.27]
Subtotal (95% CI)		**265**		**259**	**100.0%**	**0.89 [0.62, 1.26]**
Total events	97		102			
Heterogeneity: $Chi^2 = 0.32$, df = 1 (P = 0.57); $I^2 = 0\%$						
Test for overall effect: Z = 0.66 (P = 0.51)						
1.1.3 Cetrolix only						
Albano 2000	34	198	19	95	26.3%	0.83 [0.44, 1.55]
Hurine 2006	17	91	17	91	17.1%	1.00 [0.47, 2.11]
Kim 2009	13	54	8	28	9.9%	0.79 [0.28, 2.22]
Kurzawa 2008	14	37	18	37	13.8%	0.64 [0.25, 1.62]
Marci 2005	4	30	0	30	0.5%	10.36 [0.53, 201.45]
Ye 2009	35	109	39	111	32.4%	0.87 [0.50, 1.53]
Subtotal (95% CI)		**519**		**392**	**100.0%**	**0.89 [0.65, 1.23]**
Total events	117		101			
Heterogeneity: $Chi^2 = 3.31$, df = 5 (P = 0.65); $I^2 = 0\%$						
Test for overall effect: Z = 0.70 (P = 0.49)						
1.1.4 Ganirelix only						
Barmat 2005	13	40	17	40	100.0%	0.65 [0.26, 1.62]
Subtotal (95% CI)		**40**		**40**	**100.0%**	**0.65 [0.26, 1.62]**
Total events	13		17			
Heterogeneity: Not applicable						
Test for overall effect: Z = 0.92 (P = 0.36)						

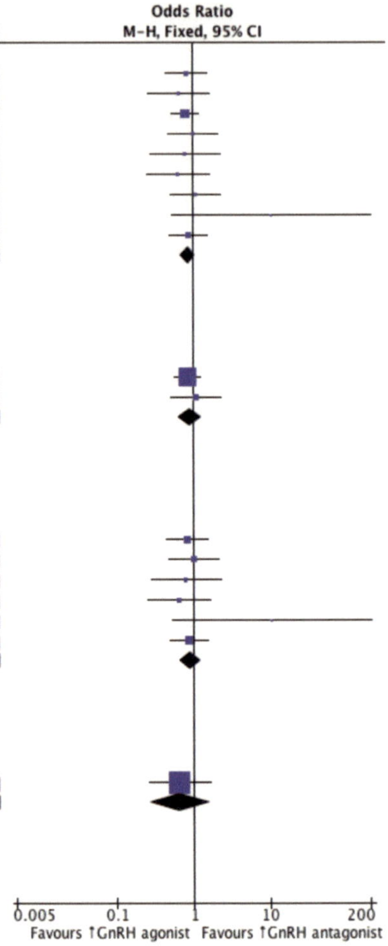

Fig. 4. Forest plot of comparison: GnRH antagonist Vs GnRH agonist live birth rate per women randomized

6.3 Changing attitudes towards diagnostics (evidence based diagnosis)

Evidence-based medicine has progressively developed as the standard approach for many diagnostic procedures. With the increasing varieties of investigating and diagnostic tools, evidence based medicine allows for the selection of the best diagnostic approach that would achieve the most reliable diagnosis with the least possible expenses, thus avoiding other less accurate and unnecessary diagnostic methods.

6.3.1 Anti-Müllerian hormone

Anti-Müllerian hormone (AMH) has become the 'molecule of the moment' in the field of Reproductive Endocrinology. Indeed, it is valuable as a means of increasing understanding of ovarian pathophysiology and for guiding clinical management across a broad range of conditions.

	GnRH antagonist		GnRH agonist			Risk Difference
Study or Subgroup	Events	Total	Events	Total	Weight	M-H, Fixed, 95% CI
1.5.1 All women						
Albano 2000	2	198	5	95	5.0%	-0.04 [-0.09, 0.00]
Badrawy 2005	2	50	2	50	2.0%	0.00 [-0.08, 0.08]
Bahceci 2005	3	73	5	75	2.9%	-0.03 [-0.10, 0.05]
Barmat 2005	0	40	0	40	1.6%	0.00 [-0.05, 0.05]
Engmann 2008 a	0	34	10	32	1.3%	-0.31 [-0.48, -0.15]
Euro Midd East 2001	4	236	1	119	6.2%	0.01 [-0.01, 0.03]
Euro Orgalutran 2000	11	486	14	244	12.8%	-0.03 [-0.07, -0.00]
Firouzabadi 2010	3	118	12	117	4.6%	-0.08 [-0.14, -0.02]
Fluker 2001	12	205	2	108	5.6%	0.04 [-0.00, 0.08]
Heijnen 2007	6	205	12	199	7.9%	-0.03 [-0.07, 0.01]
Hohmann 2003	1	97	0	45	2.4%	0.01 [-0.03, 0.05]
Hsieh 2008	3	86	2	58	2.7%	0.00 [-0.06, 0.06]
Hurine 2006	2	91	3	91	3.6%	-0.01 [-0.06, 0.04]
Hwang 2004	2	27	2	29	1.1%	0.01 [-0.13, 0.14]
Karimzadeh 2010	0	121	6	122	4.8%	-0.05 [-0.09, -0.01]
Kurzawa 2008	0	37	2	37	1.5%	-0.05 [-0.14, 0.03]
Kyono 2005	2	126	6	66	3.4%	-0.08 [-0.15, -0.00]
Lainas 2007	3	26	20	52	1.4%	-0.27 [-0.45, -0.09]
Lainas 2010	5	110	6	110	4.3%	-0.01 [-0.07, 0.05]
Lee 2005	3	40	2	20	1.0%	-0.03 [-0.18, 0.13]
Lin 2006	1	60	3	60	2.4%	-0.03 [-0.10, 0.03]
Moraloglu 2008	2	45	4	48	1.8%	-0.04 [-0.14, 0.06]
Moshin 2007	0	25	1	24	1.0%	-0.04 [-0.15, 0.07]
Olivennes 2000	4	126	4	43	2.5%	-0.06 [-0.15, 0.03]
Rombauts 2006	5	234	6	117	6.1%	-0.03 [-0.07, 0.01]
Serafini 2003	1	49	1	28	1.4%	-0.02 [-0.09, 0.06]
Tehraninejad 2010	0	45	15	47	1.8%	-0.32 [-0.45, -0.18]
Xavier 2005	4	66	1	65	2.6%	0.05 [-0.02, 0.11]
Ye 2009	3	109	2	111	4.3%	0.01 [-0.03, 0.05]
Subtotal (95% CI)		**3165**		**2252**	**100.0%**	**-0.03 [-0.05, -0.02]**
Total events	84		149			
Heterogeneity: Chi² = 86.65, df = 28 (P < 0.00001); I² = 68%						
Test for overall effect: Z = 5.96 (P < 0.00001)						
1.5.2 Regular population						
Albano 2000	2	198	5	95	6.0%	-0.04 [-0.09, 0.00]
Badrawy 2005	2	50	2	50	2.3%	0.00 [-0.08, 0.08]
Barmat 2005	0	40	0	40	1.9%	0.00 [-0.05, 0.05]
Euro Midd East 2001	4	236	1	119	7.3%	0.01 [-0.01, 0.03]
Euro Orgalutran 2000	11	486	14	244	15.1%	-0.03 [-0.07, -0.00]
Firouzabadi 2010	3	118	12	117	5.4%	-0.08 [-0.14, -0.02]
Fluker 2001	12	205	2	108	6.6%	0.04 [-0.00, 0.08]
Heijnen 2007	6	205	12	199	9.4%	-0.03 [-0.07, 0.01]
Hohmann 2003	1	97	0	45	2.9%	0.01 [-0.03, 0.05]
Hsieh 2008	3	86	2	58	3.2%	0.00 [-0.06, 0.06]
Hurine 2006	2	91	3	91	4.2%	-0.01 [-0.06, 0.04]
Karimzadeh 2010	0	121	6	122	5.6%	-0.05 [-0.09, -0.01]
Kyono 2005	2	126	6	66	4.0%	-0.08 [-0.15, -0.00]
Lee 2005	3	40	2	20	1.2%	-0.03 [-0.18, 0.13]
Lin 2006	1	60	3	60	2.8%	-0.03 [-0.10, 0.03]
Moraloglu 2008	2	45	4	48	2.2%	-0.04 [-0.14, 0.06]
Olivennes 2000	4	126	4	43	3.0%	-0.06 [-0.15, 0.03]
Rombauts 2006	5	234	6	117	7.2%	-0.03 [-0.07, 0.01]
Serafini 2003	1	49	1	28	1.7%	-0.02 [-0.09, 0.06]
Xavier 2005	4	66	1	65	3.0%	0.05 [-0.02, 0.11]
Ye 2009	3	109	2	111	5.1%	0.01 [-0.03, 0.05]
Subtotal (95% CI)		**2788**		**1846**	**100.0%**	**-0.02 [-0.03, -0.01]**
Total events	71		88			
Heterogeneity: Chi² = 35.97, df = 20 (P = 0.02); I² = 44%						
Test for overall effect: Z = 3.75 (P = 0.0002)						
1.5.3 Women with PCOS						
Bahceci 2005	3	73	5	75	19.1%	-0.03 [-0.10, 0.05]
Engmann 2008 a	0	34	10	32	8.5%	-0.31 [-0.48, -0.15]
Hwang 2004	2	27	2	29	7.2%	0.01 [-0.13, 0.14]
Kurzawa 2008	0	37	2	37	9.6%	-0.05 [-0.14, 0.03]
Lainas 2007	3	26	20	52	9.0%	-0.27 [-0.45, -0.09]
Lainas 2010	5	110	6	110	28.4%	-0.01 [-0.07, 0.05]
Moshin 2007	0	25	1	24	6.3%	-0.04 [-0.15, 0.07]
Tehraninejad 2010	0	45	15	47	11.9%	-0.32 [-0.45, -0.18]
Subtotal (95% CI)		**377**		**406**	**100.0%**	**-0.10 [-0.14, -0.07]**
Total events	13		61			
Heterogeneity: Chi² = 39.00, df = 7 (P < 0.00001); I² = 82%						
Test for overall effect: Z = 5.39 (P < 0.00001)						

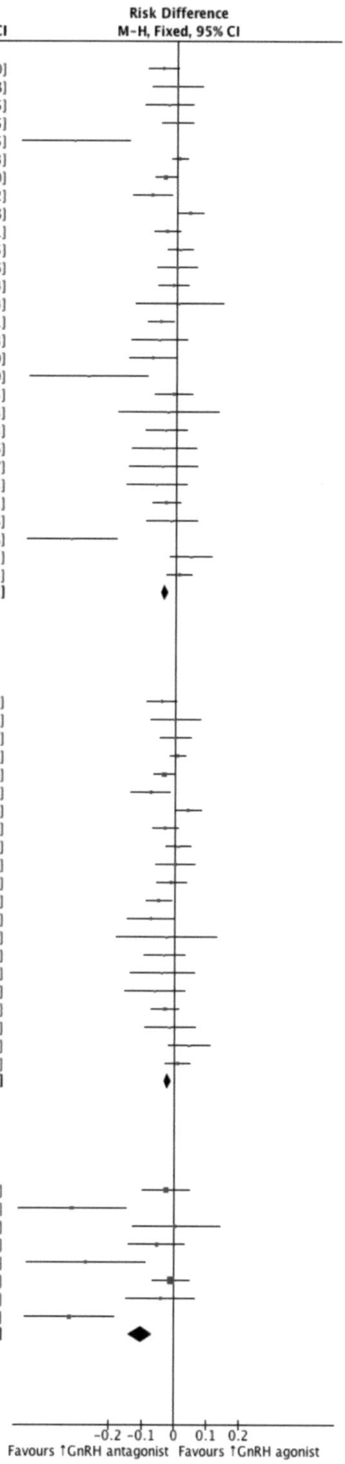

Test for subgroup differences: Chi² = 16.94, df = 2 (P = 0.0002), I² = 88.2%

Fig. 5. GnRH antagonist vs GnRH agonist ovarian hyperstimulation per women randomised

In a cross-sectional study by La Marca *et al.*, 2010, AMH was measured in 277 healthy females (aged 18–50 years) by commercial enzyme-linked immunosorbent assay. Serum AMH concentrations show a progressive decline with female ageing. The age-related changes in AMH were best fitted by a polynomial function. Mean AMH concentrations were not modified by past use of oral contraceptive and were independent of parity of women. Age-specific normative values for circulating AMH concentration were established. AMH concentrations seem to be independent of the reproductive history of the patient (La Marca *et al.*, 2010).

AMH plays a basic role as a prognostic marker in women undergoing ovarian stimulation protocols and can predict an excessive response to ovarian stimulation (Broer *et al.*, 2010).

7. Conclusions

Evidence Based Medicine is currently changing our daily practice in obstetrics and gynecology towards achieving better health to women and mothers all over the world. The best evidence can be extracted from clinically relevant research that answers a clinical question using sound methodology.

Our paradigms in the fields of diagnosis, interventions and therapeutics have exhibited some of the progress that has been performed throughout the last years. There is an increasing necessity for systematically reviewing, appraising and using clinical research findings to shift our practice towards an evidence based one. Evidence-based practice requires a clear view of the evidence combined with wise integration of this information with other knowledge and experience in clinical decision making.

Evidence based medicine has been adopted, alongside health economics, and has been promoted as the gold standard tool for advancement and provision of health services in obstetrics and gynecology. Thus, a keen and sincere physician should be seeking evidence based medicine and integrating evidence based practice to deliver a higher level of health service to his patients.

In a domain full of controversies as that of the obstetrics and gynecology, it is crucial to consider what the evidence says and exert every effort to integrate this evidence into practice as this will be the surest way that a patient will receive safe and effective up to date health service.

Drawing examples on evidence based medicine is endless and can not be fulfilled completely in this context however, we aimed to draw the light on the role of evidence based medicine in changing attitudes in our routine daily practice by demonstrating some important examples that would emphasize that role.

8. References

Abou-Setta AM, Wahba A, Madkour W, Sharif K & Al-Inany HG. Preimplantation genetic screening for aneuploidies: A systematic review and meta-analysis. *EBWHJ* 2011; 1(2): 43-50.

Al-Inany H & Aboulghar M. Gonadotrophin-releasing hormone antagonists for assisted conception. *Cochrane Database Syst. Rev.* 4, CD001750 (2001).

Al-Inany H & Aboulghar M. Gonadotrophin-releasing hormone antagonists for assisted conception. *Cochrane Database Syst. Rev.* 4, CD001750 (2003).

Al-Inany HG, Abou-Setta AM & Aboulghar M. Gonadotrophin-releasing hormone antagonists for assisted conception. *Cochrane Database Syst. Rev.* 3, CD001750 (2006).

Al-Inany H, Wahba A & Peitsidis P. Changing attitudes in ovarian stimulation. *Womens Health (Lond Engl)*. 2011; Sep;7(5):505-7.

Al-Inany HG, Youssef MA, Aboulghar M *et al.* GnRH antagonists are safer than agonists: an update of a Cochrane review. *Hum. Reprod. Update* 2011; 17(4): 435.

Asuncion M, Calvo RM, San Millan JL, Sancho J, Avila S & Escobar-Morreale HF. A prospective study of the prevalence of the polycystic ovary syndrome in unselected Caucasian women from Spain. *J Clin Endocrinol Metab* 2000; 85:2434–2438.

Batukan C & Baysal B: Metformin improves ovulation and pregnancy rates in patients with polycystic ovary syndrome. *Arch Gynecol Obstet* 2001; 265:124.

Bennett RJ, Sackett DL, Haynes RB & Neufeld VR. *A controlled trial of teaching critical appraisal of the clinical literature to medical students. JAMA* 1987;257:2451–4.

Broer SL, Dolleman M, Opmeer BC, Fauser BC, Mol BW & Broekmans FJM. "AMH and AFC as predictors of excessive response in controlled ovarian hyperstimulation: a meta-analysis". *Human Reproduction Update* .2010. 17 (1): 46.

Caglar GS, Asimakopoulos B, Nikolettos N, Diedrich K & Al-Hasani S. Preimplantation genetic diagnosis for aneuploidy screening in repeated implantation failure. *Reprod Biomed Online* 2005;10: 381-8.

Costello MF, Chapman M & Conway U. A systematic review and meta-analysis of randomised controlled trials on metformin coadministration during gonadotropin ovulation induction or IVF in women with polycystic ovary syndrome. *Hum Reprod* 2006; 21: 1387-99.

Cochrane A. Effectiveness and efficiency. Random reflections on health services. The Nuffield Provincial Hospitals Trust; 1972.

Chalmers I, Hetherington J, Newdick M, Mutch L, Grant A, Enkin M, et al. The Oxford database of perinatal trials: developing a register of published reports of controlled trials. Controlled Clinical Trials 1986;7:306e24.

Delhanty JD, Harper JC, Ao A, Handyside AH & Winston RM. Multicolour FISH detects frequent chromosomal mosaicism and chaotic division in normal preimplantation embryos from fertile patients. *Hum Genet* 1997;99:755-60.

Diamanti-Kandarakis E, Kouli C, Tsianateli T, et al: Therapeutic effects of metformin on insulin resistance and hyperandrogenism in polycystic ovary syndrome. *Eur J Endocrinol* 1998; 138:269.

Dodd JM & Crowther CA. Cochrane reviews in pregnancy: the role of perinatal randomized trials and systematic reviews in establishing evidence. Semin Fetal Neonatal Med. 2006 Apr;11(2):97-103. Epub 2006 Jan 18. Review

Donoghue D, Bawden K, Cartwright D, Darlow B, Henderson- Smart D & Lancaster P. The report of the Australian and New Zealand Neonatal Network, 2000. Sydney: ANZNN; 2002.

Dorval M, Vallee MH, Plante M, *et al.* Effect of the Women's Health Initiative study publication on hormone replacement therapy use among women who have undergone BRCA1/2 testing. *Cancer Epidemiol Biomark and Preven* 2007; 16: 157-60.

Enkin M, Keirse M & Chalmers IE. A guide to effective care in pregnancy and childbirth. Oxford: Oxford University Press;1989.

Essah PA, Apridonidze T, Iuorno MJ, et al: Effects of short-term and long-term metformin treatment on menstrual cyclicity in women with polycystic ovary syndrome. *Fertil Steril* 2006; 86:230.

Felberbaum RE, Reissmann T, Kuper W *et al.* Preserved pituitary response under ovarian stimulation with hMG and GnRH-antagonists (Cetrorelix) in women with tubal infertility. *Eur. J. Obstet. Gynecol. Reprod. Biol.* 1995; 61(2): 151–155 .

Gianaroli L, Magli MC, Ferraretti AP, Tabanelli C, Trengia V, Farfalli V et al. The beneficial effects of preimplantation genetic diagnosis for aneuploidy support extensive clinical application. Reprod Biomed Online 2005;10: 633-40.

Grimshaw, Ward, Eccles (2001). *Oxford Handbook of Public Health.* Watt (2002) *Lancet*

Guyatt G & Rennie DE. Users' Guide to the Medical Literature. A manual for evidence based practice. JAMA and Archives Journals, The American Medical Associations; 2002.

Hannah ME, Hannah WJ, Hewson SA, Hodnett ED, Saigal S & Willan AR. Planned caesarean section versus planned vaginal birth for breech presentation at term: a randomised multicentre trial. Term Breech Trial Collaborative Group. *Lancet.* 2000 Oct 21;356(9239):1375-83.

Harper JC, Coonen E, Handyside AH, Winston RM, Hopman AH & Delhanty JD. Mosaicism of autosomes and sex chromosomes in morphologically normal, monospermic preimplantation human embryos. Prenat Diagn 1995;15:41-9.

Haas DA, Carr BR, Attia GR: Effects of metformin on body mass index, menstrual cyclicity, and ovulation induction in women with polycystic ovary syndrome. *Fertil Steril* 2003; 79:469.

Haynes RB, Devereaux PJ & Guyatt GH. "Clinical expertise in the era of evidence-based medicine and patient choice", *ACP Journal Club,* 2002; 136 (2): A11-14.

Hersh A, Stefanick M, & Stafford R. National use of postmenopausal hormone therapy: annual trends and response to recent evidence. *JAMA* 2004; 291:47-53.

Hull MG. Epidemiology of infertility and polycystic ovarian disease: endocrinological and demographic studies. *Gynecol Endocrinol* 1987; 1:235–245

Kahraman S, Benkhalifa M, Donmez E, Biricik A, Sertyel S, Findikli N et al. The results of aneuploidy screening in 276 couples undergoing assisted reproductive techniques. *Prenat Diagn* 2004;24:307-11.

Kaushik V & Gudgeon C. Caesarean for breech: A paradigm shift? *Aust NZ J Obstet Gynaecol.*2003 43, 298-301.

Knochenhauer ES, Key TJ, Kahsar-Miller M, Waggoner W, Boots LR, Azziz R. Prevalence of the polycystic ovary syndrome in unselected black and white women of the southeastern United States: a prospective study. *J Clin Endocrinol Metab* 1998; 83:3078–3082.

Kosmas IP, Tatsioni A, Fatemi HM, Kolibianakis EM, Tournaye H & Devroey P. Human chorionic gonadotropin administration vs. luteinizing monitoring for intrauterine insemination timing, after administration of clomiphene citrate: a meta-analysis. *Fertil Steril.* 2007 Mar; 87(3):607-12.

Kyrgiou M,Koliopoulos G,Martin-Hirsch P,Arbyn M,Prendiville M, & Paraskevaidis E. Obstetric outcomes after conservative treatment for intraepithelial or early invasive cervical lesions: systematic review and meta-analysis. *Lancet.* 2006;367(9509):489-98.

La Marca A, Sighinolfi G, Giulini S, Traglia M, Argento C, Sala C, Masciullo C, Volpe A & Toniolo D. Normal serum concentrations of anti-Müllerian hormone in women with regular menstrual cycles. *Reprod Biomed Online.* 2010 Oct;21(4):463-9.

Laudański T & Pierzyński P. Evidence-based medicine and medical databases in obstetrics and gynecology. *Ginekologia Polska* 2000; *71*(1): 39-44

Legro RS, Barnhart HX, Schlaff WD, Carr BR, Diamond MP, Carson SA, Steinkampf MP, Coutifaris C, McGovern PG, Cataldo NA, Gosmon GG, et al. Cooperative Multicenter Reproductive Medicine Network. (2007) Clomiphene, metformin, or both for infertility in the polycystic ovary syndrome. *N Engl J Med* 2007;356:551-566.

Lindsay R, Aitken JM, Anderson JD, et al. Long-term prevention of postmenopausal osteoporosis by oestrogen. *Lancet* 1976;i:1038–1041.

Magli MC, Gianaroli L & Ferraretti AP. Chromosomal abnormalities in embryos. *Mol Cell Endocrinol* 2001;183 Suppl 1:S29-34.

Majumdar S, Almasi E & Stafford R. Promotion and prescribing of hormone therapy after report of harm by the Women's Health Initiative. *JAMA* 2004; 292:1983-88.

Mansour RT & Aboulghar MA. Optimizing the embryo transfer technique. Hum Reprod 2002;17:1149-53

Moll E, Bossuyt PM, Korevaar JC, Lambalk CB & van der Veen F. Effect of clomifene citrate plus metformin and clomifene citrate plus placebo on induction of ovulation in women with newly diagnosed polycystic ovary syndrome: randomised double blind clinical trial. *BMJ* 2006; 332:1485.

Munne S, Sandalinas M, Escudero T, Velilla E, Walmsley R, Sadowy S et al. Improved implantation after preimplantation genetic diagnosis of aneuploidy. Reprod Biomed Online 2003;7: 91-7.

Munne S, Bahce M, Sandalinas M, Escudero T, Marquez C, Velilla E et al. Differences in chromosome susceptibility to aneuploidy and survival to first trimester. Reprod Biomed Online 2004;8: 81-90.

Neveu N, Granger L, St-Michel P, et al: Comparison of clomiphene citrate, metformin, or the combination of both for first-line ovulation induction and achievement of pregnancy in 154 women with polycystic ovary syndrome. *Fertil Steril* 2007; 87(1):113.

Piltonen T, Morin-Papunen L, Koivunen R, Perheentupa A, Ruokonen A & Tapanainen JS. Serum anti-Mullerian hormone levels remain high until late reproductive age and decrease during metformin therapy in women with polycystic ovary syndrome. *Hum Reprod* 2005; 20: 1820-6.

Phipps H, Roberts CL, Nassar N, Rayes-Greenow CH, Peat B, and Hutton EK. The management of breech pregnancies in Australia and New Zealand. *Aust NZ J Obstet Gynaecol* 2003; 43: 294-297.

Rizk B & Smitz J. Ovarian hyperstimulation syndrome after superovulation using GnRH agonists for IVF and related procedures. *Hum. Reprod.* 1992; 7(3): 320–327.

Rizk B & Aboulghar MA. Classification, pathophysiology and management of ovarian hyperstimulation syndrome. In: *A Textbook of In Vitro Fertilization and Assisted*

Reproduction. Brinsden P (Ed.). The Parthenon Publishing Group, New York, NY, USA (1999).

Rosenberg W & Donald A. Evidence based medicine: an approach to clinical problem-solving. *BMJ* 1995; 310: 1122–1126.

Sackett DL, Rosenberg WM, Gray JA, Haynes RB & Richardson WS. Evidence based medicine: what it is and what it isn't. *BMJ* 1996. 312: 71

Sackett DL. Evidence-based medicine. *Semin Perinatol*. 1997 Feb;21(1):3-5

Sackett D, Richardson WS, Rosenberg W & Haynes RB. *Evidence-Based Medicine*: How to Practice and Teach EBM. London: Churchill Livingstone, 1997

Sackett DL, Straus SE, Richardson WS, Rosenberg W & Haynes RB. Evidence-based medicine; how to practice and teach EBM. 2nd ed. Edinburgh: Churchill Livingstone, 2000: 82-4.

Sermon K, Moutou C, Harper J, Geraedts J, Scriven P, Wilton L et al. ESHRE PGD Consortium data collection IV: May-December 2001. *Hum Reprod* 2005;20:19-34.

Shin JH, Flaynes RB & Johnston ME. *Effect of problem-based, self-directed undergraduate education on life-long learning. Can Med Assoc J 1993;148:969–76.*

Stampfer MJ, Colditz GA, Willett WC, et al. Postmenopausal estrogen therapy and cardiovascular disease: ten-year follow-up from the nurses' health study. *N Engl J Med* 1991;325:756–762.

The Cochrane Library. 2005; Issue 3. www3.interscience.wiley.com.

Tang T, Glanville J, Orsi N, Barth JH & Balen AH. The use of metformin for women with PCOS undergoing IVF treatment. *Hum Reprod* 2006; 21: 1416-25.

Wilton L. Preimplantation genetic diagnosis for aneuploidy screening in early human embryos: a review. *Prenat Diagn* 2002; 22: 512-8.

Wright RC. Reduction of perinatal mortality and morbidity in breech delivery through routine use of cesarean section. *Obstetrics and Gynecology* 1959; 14(6): 758-763.

Rossouw JE, Anderson GL, Prentice RL, LaCroix AZ, Kooperberg C, Stefanick ML, Jackson RD, Beresford SA, Howard BV, Johnson KC, Kotchen JM, Ockene J; Writing Group for the Women's Health Initiative Investigators: Risks and benefits of estrogen plus progestin in healthy postmenopausal women. Principal results from the Women's Health Initiative randomized controlled trial. *JAMA* 2002; 28:321-333.

8

Evidence-Based Cervical Cancer Screening: The Modern Evolution of the Pap Smear

Justin Lappen[1] and Dana R. Gossett[2]
[1]*Case Western Reserve University School of Medicine, Cleveland, OH,*
[2]*Northwestern University Feinberg School of Medicine, Chicago IL*
USA

1. Introduction

The Papanicolou screen ("Pap smear") was developed in 1928 by Dr. George Papanicolaou for the identification of cervical cancers. It became widely known after his publication in 1941 and widely used in clinical practice in the 1950s; it is now the most commonly performed cancer screening test world-wide (1). This has been one of the most successful cancer screening techniques in modern medicine, and in the United States rates of cervical cancer have decreased by almost 80% since the 1950s (2,3). Pap smear screening has been widely embraced by physicians and women alike, and is considered a critical part of the routine health care of women. However, up to 20% of American women do not receive regular Pap smears, and in developing countries without the complex resources required to process and read Pap specimens, screening remains a challenge (4). Among women with cervical cancer in the U.S., at least 60% did not have appropriate Pap surveillance prior to their diagnoses (5).

In the decades since the initial development of the Pap smear, our understanding of the pathophysiology of cervical cancer has evolved considerably. The occurrence of pre-malignant cervical lesions, now referred to as cervical dysplasia, was recognized as early at the 1940s (6). During the 1970s and 1980s, the human Papilloma virus (HPV) was identified within cervical lesions (7, 8). As early as 1976, Dr. Harald zur Hausen and colleagues postulated a role for the HPV in cervical oncogenesis, and his subsequent work isolating oncogenic HPV strains and elucidating the oncogenic process earned him the Nobel Prize in Medicine in 2008 (9-11).

The discoveries of premalignant cervical lesions and the role of HPV in cervical dysplasias and cancers have also enabled physicians to gradually refine the use of Pap smear screening. As a result, the number of women who need Pap smears, and the frequency at which they are recommended, has changed significantly over the last several years. However, dissemination of the newest guidelines has been met with some resistance both from women and their physicians.

In this article, we will review these advancements and the current evidence about the modern use of Pap smears and HPV screening, the evidence leading to the new recommendations and some barriers to their full implementation.

2. Fundamentals of screening for disease

Screening can be defined as the effort to identify asymptomatic disease or disease precursors through examinations or tests applied rapidly to an appropriate segment of the population. Screening tests delineate patients who appear well and have a disease from those who do not have a disease. Numerous examples of screening tests exist in clinical practice as a part of primary or secondary prevention, including blood pressure measurements, serum cholesterol measurements, pap tests, and colonoscopy. Importantly, screening tests are not intended to be diagnostic. A positive screening test requires follow-up and commitment to further investigation.

A successful and appropriate screening test depends on numerous criteria, which cluster in to three general categories delineated by Katz: disease-specific criteria, test-specific criteria, and society or system-criteria (Table 1) (12). All of the factors listed in Table 1 impact the potential benefits of screening programs both to individual patients and populations. Disease screening would be unjustified if the burden of disease is insignificant or if treatment outcomes are no different between asymptomatic cases diagnosed at an early stage and symptomatic cases diagnosed at later stage. If an effective treatment for a disease is not available, screening and early detection confers no benefit to patients. Disease prevalence, discussed in detail below, is integral to screening programs as screening for extremely rare conditions would not be cost-effective or accurate given that false-positive tests may outnumber true-positive results. The screening test itself must be convenient, acceptable, safe, and cost-effective for patients. An ideal screening test should take only a

Disease-specific

- Condition must have significant burden on health (morbidity, mortality, suffering)
- Disease detectable in asymptomatic state
- Natural history of disease modifiable with treatment
- Early, effective treatment available
- Appropriate prevalence: not too rare or too common

Test-specific

- Highly sensitive to reliably identify disease cases
- Highly specific to minimize false positives
- Cost-effective
- Test is safe, convenient, and acceptable to patients

Society/System-specific

- Confirmatory, diagnostic testing readily available for screen positive
- Effective treatment readily available for confirmed cases
- Screening program cost-effective for population

Adapted from Katz DL, Fundamentals of screening: the art and science of looking for trouble, Sage Publications, London, 2001 (reference 12).

Table 1. Characteristics of an Appropriate Screening Test

few minutes to perform, require minimal preparation by the patient, and be inexpensive. Additionally, given that screening programs require a significant commitment of resources, they should be cost-effective and confer benefit on a population or societal level. As described further in this chapter, screening for cervical cancer exemplifies an ideal screening test by meeting all of the aforementioned criteria.

Importantly, a successful screening program is dependent upon the various characteristics of the screening test, and an understanding of these principals is fundamental to providers and public health officials. Sensitivity and specificity are characteristics inherent to a test and are independent of disease prevalence. Sensitivity is the probability that if the disease is present, the test is positive. Mathematically, the numerator is the number of subjects with a disease who have a positive test and the denominator is the total number of subjects with a disease. A test with high sensitivity effectively identifies subjects with disease and infrequently misses true cases (low false negative rate). Specificity is the probability that if a disease is absent, the test is negative. Mathematically, the numerator is the number of subjects without a disease who also have a negative test, and the denominator is the total number of subjects without disease. Tests with high specificity infrequently identify subjects as having disease when they do not (low false positive rate). Given that screening tests must identify disease in asymptomatic patients where the prevalence is usually low (even in high risk groups), a good screening test must have high sensitivity as to not miss the few cases of disease present. Additionally, the sensitivity must remain high in the early stages of disease. A test that demonstrates high sensitivity only in late-stage disease, where treatment may be less effective, will not provide clinical utility. Good screening tests should also have high specificity to reduce the number of false positive results which require follow-up evaluation or intervention.

The calculation of sensitivity and specificity for screening tests are determined in a manner similar to that of diagnostic tests, however one major difference deserves mention. The sensitivity and specificity of diagnostic tests are based on comparisons between the test results and a different test (the reference or "gold standard"). For a screening test, the "gold standard" for detecting disease includes both another test and a period of follow-up. Additional testing is routinely administered to those who have positive screening tests for confirmation (differentiation of true and false-positive results). However, a period of follow-up is necessary for all negative results to differentiate subjects with true and false-negative tests. This characteristic is particularly important in cancer screening, where cancers discovered during the period of follow-up (interval cancers) occur. Choosing the appropriate duration of follow-up may impact the sensitivity and specificity of the test, which overestimates sensitivity if the follow-up period is too short and underestimates sensitivity if the follow-up period is too long. (13)

Positive and negative predictive values (PPV, NPV) also represent important characteristics of screening tests. PPV represents the probability that a subject with a positive test has a disease. The numerator is the number of subjects with disease who have a positive test and the denominator is the number of subjects with a positive test. Conversely, NPV represents the probability that subject with a negative test does not have disease. The numerator is the number of subjects without disease who have a negative test and the denominator is the number of subjects with a negative test. The predictive values depend on disease prevalence within a population. For a test with a given sensitivity and specificity, as prevalence rises the PPV of a test increases and the NPV decreases. Conversely, as prevalence falls, the PPV decreases and the NPV increases. This observation has important implications for screening tests, where the disease prevalence is generally low. Therefore, most screening tests have low PPV and high NPV (despite high sensitivity and specificity). Clinically, this implies that providers offering screening tests to their patients must accept the fact that many patients will screen positive and not truly have disease; however, these patients still require follow-up evaluation and testing.

3. Biases and pitfalls of screening programs

Instinctively, screening for disease has apparent benefits. However, given that no test in medicine is perfect, widespread adoption of screening tests prior proving their benefit can become problematic. Therefore, prior to implementing population-wide screening programs, a test should be subject to careful study. Similar to any intervention in medicine, the most rigorous means of establishing the efficacy of a treatment or intervention is with a randomized controlled trial. However, many years and large numbers of patients are required to establish the efficacy of a preventative intervention or screening test. For example, a study demonstrating that early treatment of colorectal cancer detected by disease screening reduced cancer-related mortality by one-third required 45,000 subjects and 13 years of follow-up surveillance (14). Therefore, a case series describing screening programs or a "clinical impressions" of the impact of screening do not suffice to establish efficacy.

Rigorous study is necessary to avoid biases specific to the study of screening programs. One such bias, lead-time bias, occurs when discovering a disease in an early stage with screening does not impact mortality rates or outcomes relative to discovering the disease later when it would typically present with symptoms. Discovering the disease early may appear beneficial by increasing "survival time". However, in reality, early detection only serves to advance diagnosis, thereby increasing the duration of time a patient has a disease. A patient living with disease for a longer period of time may be subject to more frequent examinations and tests as well as increased anxiety from a longer time with knowledge of disease.

Another type of bias present in screening programs is length-time bias. Length-time bias is a type of selection bias that occurs when outcomes appear better in a screened population of subjects due to the fact that diseases with a favorable prognosis are more readily discovered with screening. This phenomenon is exemplified by cancer screening, where slow-growing lesions are diagnosed more readily than rapidly-growing lesions due to a longer pre-clinical, asymptomatic period. Given that slow-growing tumors generally have a better prognosis than rapidly-growing tumors, screening programs generally discover slow-growing tumors with inherently more favorable prognoses. Therefore, while mortality rates for cancers discovered through screening may be more favorable, screening is not truly protective in this setting.

Lastly, compliance bias can occur in studying the efficacy of screening programs. Compliance, the degree to which patients follow or adhere to medical advice, may impact studies of disease screening as compliant patients tend to have better prognoses independent of screening. For example, studies that compare disease outcomes between subjects who volunteer for screening and those that do not may demonstrate improved outcome, however this improvement may be secondary to higher compliance amongst volunteers rather than any benefit conferred by the screening program. Therefore, to effectively evaluate the impact of any screening test or program, randomized trials with concurrent screening and control groups must be conducted to minimize the introduction of length-time and compliance bias. By following studied populations with mortality rates, rather than survival rates, lead-time bias can be avoided.

Screening programs also have the potential to produce significant adverse effects in a screened population, which highlights another critical reason to rigorously study screening tests prior to their widespread application. Adverse effects range from discomfort produced from the test itself to false-positive test results to overdiagnosis. In effective screening programs, false-positive results account for a minority of all test results. However, false-positive results can still have a substantial impact on a large number of patients by producing anxiety and the discomfort and cost of additional follow-up tests. Given that screening tests are often repeated in intervals, each repeat screen is subject to further false-positive results. Additionally, the negative impact of overdiagnosis cannot be overstated. While the underlying presumption in cancer screening is that earlier detection translates into improved outcomes, recent evidence has challenged this thesis. In a recent editorial, Welch reviewed the impact of a 10-year course of screening mammography on 2500 women in the US at age 50 (15). While one breast cancer-related death would be prevented by mammography, up to 1000 women will have at least one false-positive result and approximately half will undergo a breast biopsy. Additionally, breast cancer will be overdiagnosed in 5-15 women who will be treated "needlessly" with surgery, chemotherapy, radiation, or a combination thereof. Therefore, even excellent screening tests are not without pitfalls.

Screening for cervical cancer exemplifies a good screening test by satisfying the aforementioned criteria described by Katz (Table 1). Cervical cancer is appropriately prevalent and has a significant disease-related morbidity and mortality. The natural history of the disease, from HPV infection to carcinoma, has been clearly established. A premalignant window for intervention exists such that treatment significantly decreases disease burden. Follow-up testing with colposcopy is generally available and effective at detecting premaligant lesions. Excision procedures reliably treat premalignant lesions and prevent progression to cancer. When utilized for screening, Pap smears have acceptable test characteristics. While reports of sensitivity and specificity vary significantly between studies, a meta-analysis demonstrated sensitivity as high as 86% and specificity as high as 100% (16). Additionally, negative predictive values have been demonstrated to be higher than 95% (17). As such, Pap screening remains one of the most significant and successful screening tests in the history of modern medicine. The remainder of this chapter provides and evidence-based assessment of Pap and HPV screening with a discussion current recommendations and controversies.

4. History of Pap screening and impact of screening on cervical cancer incidence and mortality

Dr. George Papanicolaou, a physician and scientist trained in Greece in the early 1900s, immigrated to the United States in 1913 seeking greater opportunities in medicine and research (Figure 1). He became acquainted with T.H. Morgan, a well-known zoologist who had already read and cited Papanicolaou's doctoral thesis in a publication. Mr. Morgan

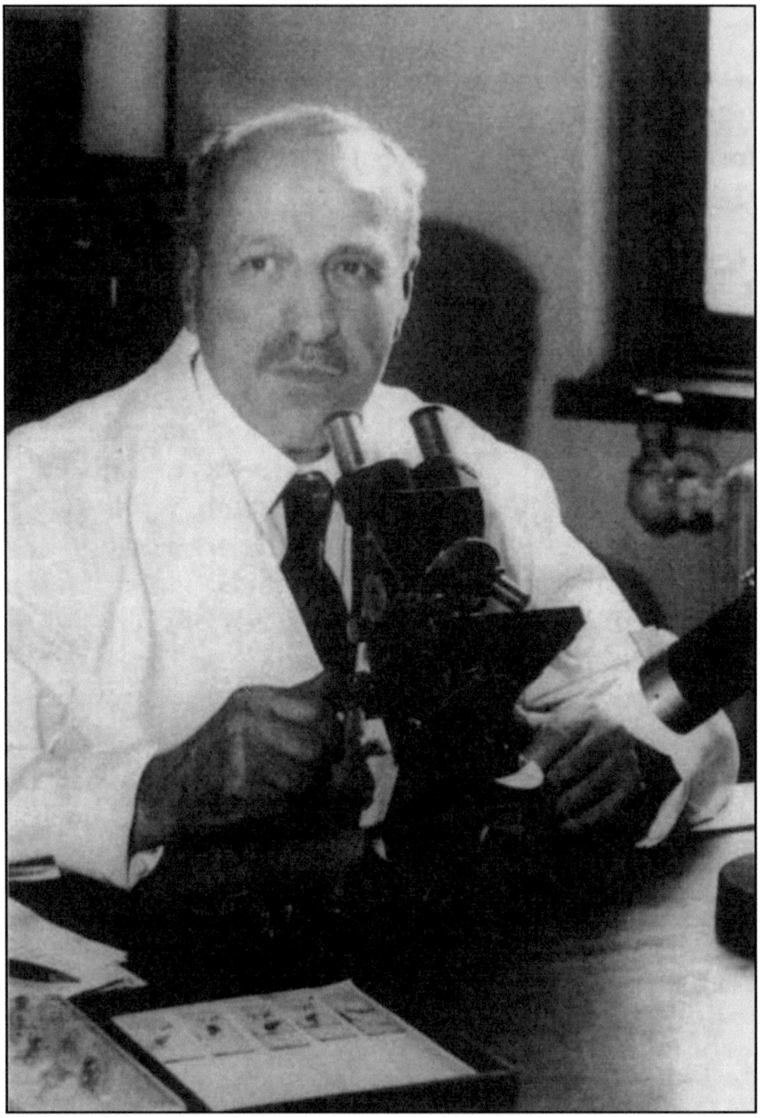

Adapted from Vilos G. Dr. George Papanicolaou and the Birth of the Pap Test. Obstetrical & Gynecological Survey. 54(8):481-483, August 1999.

Fig. 1. Dr. George Papanicolaou

recommended Papanicolaou for a part time position as a technician in the pathology department at New York Hospital. His scientific mind impressed the department and shortly thereafter he was appointed as an assistant professor in the anatomy department at Cornell Medical School. His research on the chromosomal basis of gender differentiation in guinea pigs led to the discovery that exfoliated cells from the vagina could predict the timing of ovulation. In his initial experiments, he used a small nasal speculum to obtain the sample and then plated slides for microscopy, noting "an impressive wealth of diverse cell forms and a sequence of distinctive cytologic pattern" (21). With this observation, he hypothesized that an analogous pattern could be appreciated in humans. Concomitantly, he began to obtain samples from his wife for further study, which represented the birth of the Pap smear. Shortly thereafter, he initiated the systematic study of exfoliated vaginal cells in women working at New York Hospital. In February 1295, he encountered a woman with an undiagnosed carcinoma of the cervix. The slide produced from her sample was recognized as cancer, and he then understood the implications of his methods on the diagnosis of cervical cancer. He confirmed his findings by recruiting other women with known cervical cancers and characterizing their cervicovaginal samples. He presented his test and findings at the Third Race Betterment Conference in Battle Creek, Michigan in January of 1928 (22).

Papanicolaou's 1928 presentation was greeted with skepticism by pathologists at the time as they felt biopsy should remain the gold standard diagnostic modality. Unfortunately, ten additional years of research was required before the Pap test was evaluated rigorously as a potential diagnostic tool. Finally, in 1939, at the urging of his department chair, Papanicolaou and fellow gynecologic pathologist Herbert F. Traut initiated a clinical trial of the Pap test. Vaginal samples were collected from all women admitted to the obstetric and gynecologic services at New York Hospital. They published their findings in the *American Journal of Obstetrics and Gynecology* in 1941, which detailed the differences between normal and malignant cells of the cervix. In this landmark publication, Papanicolaou proposed his technique as a simple, inexpensive means to test large numbers of women and diagnose cancer at an earlier stage which would be more amenable to treatment (1).

Shortly after the publication of this manuscript, his technique started to gain more widespread acceptance including the support of the National Cancer Institute and the American Cancer Society (ACS). In 1948, the ACS held the first interdisciplinary conference to promote the "Pap" test (23). In the late 1940s and early 1950s, community-based projects were undertaken to explore the feasibility and acceptance of screening large proportions of the population as well as to evaluate the impact of screening on cancer incidence and mortality. Screening programs in Ohio, Tennessee, and Kentucky all demonstrated increases in the detection of carcinoma in situ and decreases in the incidence of invasive carcinoma. For example, in the study from Kentucky, over 90% of the female population in the greater Louisville area was screened at least once during an 11 year period and the rate of cervical cancer declined by 32% (24-26).

With local and regional programs demonstrating benefit, the ACS promoted a national effort and campaign for screening. In 1957, the ACS initiated a campaign for annual, universal screening called the "Uterine Cancer Year". The American College of Obstetricians and Gynecologists followed with recommendations for cervical cytologic screening in their first and second editions of the Manual of Standards in Obstetric-Gynecologic Practice, published in 1959 and 1965 respectively (27). At that point, the framework was in place for the incorporation of Pap screening into standard gynecologic practice.

The aforementioned community-based evaluations established that cervical cytologic screening was acceptable to large populations of women. Importantly, these evaluations also demonstrated a consistent decrease in cervical cancer incidence and mortality in each community where screening was introduced. Interestingly, however, no randomized clinical trials of cervical cytology assessment with Pap screening have been performed to date.

Therefore, while a true causal relationship may never be formally established, a consistent association of screening with a reduction in cervical cancer burden provides convincing evidence of the impact of the Pap test.

The international epidemiology of cervical cancer further supports a direct correlation between screening programs and decreased cancer incidence and mortality. Prior to the widespread adoption of screening programs in developed countries, incidence rates of cervical cancer were similar to those found in developing countries today (28). Currently, however, marked disparities exist between the incidence of cervical cancer as well as cervical cancer-related mortality between the developed and developing world (Figure 2). Due to widespread implementation of cervical cancer screening programs in the developed world, cervical cancer has become one of the least common malignancies impacting women. In the United States in 2007, approximately 12,000 women were diagnosed with cervical cancer and 4000 died from the disease. Additionally, as noted by the NCI Surveillance Epidemiology and End Results (SEER) data, the incidence and mortality rate for cervical cancer continues to decline at 2.6% per year and 0.6% per year respectively (data available through 2008) (29, 30). Worldwide, however, the incidence of cervical cancer is approximately 500,000 cases per year with over 250,000 cancer-related deaths (31). According to the World Health Organization, over 80% of cervical cancer-related deaths occur in the developing world, and the lack of access to screening and prevention programs represents the primary reason for the enormous disparity between resource-rich and resource-poor nations (32). Additionally, even in countries with adequate screening programs, poor women suffer a disproportionate share of the burden of disease, with incidence rates

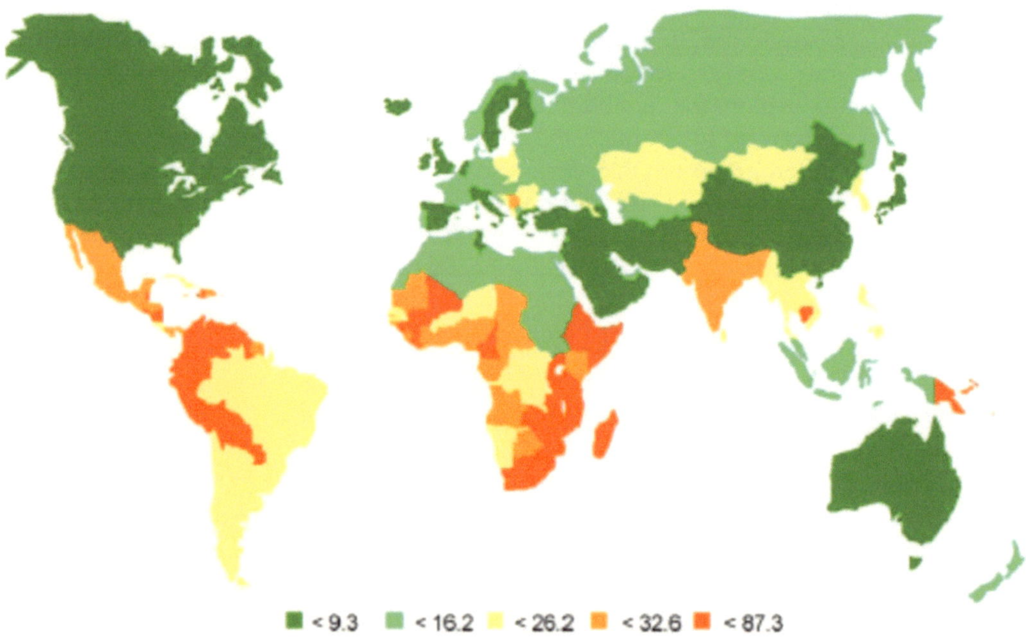

Adapted from: Sankaranarayanan R, Ferlay J. Worldwide burden of gyaecological cancer: the size of the problem. Best Pract Res Clinc Obstet Gynaecol. 2006;20:207-225.

Fig. 2. Age-standardized incidence rates of cervical cancer per 100,000 women

approximately two-fold higher than more affluent women (28). Cervical cancer does not make the list of the ten most incident or lethal cancers in the United States. However, cervical cancer remains the second leading cause of cancer-related female mortality worldwide (29, 32). It is therefore a substantial public health challenge despite the presence of an effective screening test. Moving forward, resources must be allocated for the development of comprehensive screening programs as well as HPV vaccination programs in the developing world.

5. HPV as the causative agent for cervical cancer

Human Papilloma viruses (HPV) were first identified in cervical cancer cells in 1947 by Pund et al, who noted "koilocytic changes" in cervical tissues (6). Subsequently, multiple investigators have elucidated that infection with HPV is the critical factor in cervical oncogenesis (7-11). There are over 120 strains of HPV, and approximately 30 strains affect the anogenital region (33). These are classified as either "low risk" or "high risk" HPV subtypes. Low risk HPV subtypes include 6, 11, 40, 42 and 43 and are associated with genital warts, but not significantly associated with cervical cancer. High risk HPV subtypes include 16, 18, 31, 33, 35, 39, 45, 51, 52, 56 and 58; these are associated with cervical dysplasia and cancer. HPV 16 accounts for approximately half of squamous cervical cancers, HPV 18 for another 10-15%, and 31, 33, 35, 52 and 58 about 2-5% each. Overall, between 95-100% of squamous cervical cancers are HPV-related (34, 35).

HPV is a family of double-stranded, circular DNA viruses. The genome codes for two oncogenic proteins, E6 and E7, that interfere with control of host cell replication. The E6 protein binds to the tumor suppressor gene, p53, and inactivates it. The E7 protein binds to the Rb tumor suppressor gene which results in loss of apoptosis and cell-cycle control. This leads to unchecked replication of infected cells, and shedding of the virus which can be passed on to new hosts. Episomal replication can lead to destabilization of host genome and aneuploidy, which in turn may promote integration of the HPV genome in fragile areas of the host DNA. Integration of HPV DNA into the host cell DNA is associated with cervical dysplasias and cancer.

HPV is transmitted by sexual contact, and in fact is the most common sexually transmitted infection in the world. Population-based studies have found that the lifetime prevalence of HPV infection is 50-80% (35). The estimated attack rate after contact with an HPV-infected partner is 66% (34). However, over 75% of HPV infections are asymptomatic, and are cleared by the host immune system within 6-24 months without clinical sequelae (34, 36-39). Most of these infections are not evident to the patient and are never detected before they are cleared. For patients with HPV that is clinically detected, approximately 70% will demonstrate viral clearance within one year, and 90% within two years. Importantly, it is *persistent* infection with high risk HPV that is associated with progressive cervical dysplasias and cervical cancer.

Screening for cervical cancer consists of cytologic screening—the Pap smear—either alone or in conjunction with HPV testing. In the following sections we will review screening strategies and the current recommendations for the use of both Pap smears and the available HPV tests.

6. Pap smear screening strategies

Pap smear screening has been considered an integral part of well-woman care for over 50 years, and both physicians and women have incorporated it into their annual routines. Because of the recognition that sexual debut put women at risk for HPV, older guidelines recommended starting Pap smear screening at coitarche, or by age 18 if coitarche had not occurred. Pap smears were performed annually throughout a woman's life, without a recommended terminus. A better understanding of the epidemiology and time course of HPV infection has allowed these long-standing recommendations to be gradually modified, in order to minimize unnecessary testing.

6.1 Adolescents and young women

When considering younger women, two points are important to bear in mind. The first is that the interval between HPV infection and a clinically detectable cervical dysplasia is months to several years. The second is that HPV is highly prevalent (up to 80%) and usually transient (without clinical sequelae) (34, 36, 39, 40). Understanding the time course initially led to an updated recommendation that women should start Pap smear screening three years after coitarche or by age 21. However, a finer understanding of both points together implies that detection of minor abnormalities in very young women is probably clinically irrelevant, because they nearly always resolve. Only 1 of 1000 women diagnosed with cervical cancer in the United States are under the age of 21, or approximately 10-12 women per year nationwide (41). Thus, current guidelines from the multiple American College of Obstetrics and Gynecology (ACOG) have been simplified to recommend initiation of Pap smear screening at age 21, regardless of the timing of sexual debut (40).

Between the ages of 21 and 29, two different possible screening strategies are recommended. Currently, ACOG recommend biennial screening for these women. The American Society for Colposcopy and Cervical Pathology (ASCCP), ACS and the United States Preventative Services Task Force (USPSTF) have recently released draft consensus guidelines which recommend Pap smear screening every 3 years in this age group (40, 42, 43).

6.2 Adult women

Starting at age 30, the recommended interval for Pap smear screening can be extended, assuming several criteria are met. First, healthy women who have reached age 30 and have had three prior consecutive normal Pap smears can then extend their Pap screening interval to every three years. Second, women who have a normal Pap smear *and* a negative high risk HPV test can then be screened every three years (see additional information in "HPV Screening Strategies", below). Women in either group are unlikely to develop a clinically significant dysplasia during the two unscreened years, and the resultant decrease in unnecessary Pap smears should translate into a significant savings to the health care system (40, 42).

There are several important caveats to extended interval screening. First, it is key that women are educated about the rationale for extended interval screening, and that they understand that their "annual exam" consists of more than their Pap smear. Women should be encouraged to have a regular physical examination even in the years when a Pap is not indicated. Second, there are a number of exclusion criteria for extended interval screening. Women with a history of moderate to severe cervical dysplasia (grades 2 or 3) are not eligible for this extended interval; they should continue annual Pap smears for at least twenty years after treatment. Other women who should continue to have annual screening include women exposed to diethylstilbesterol (DES), women on immunosuppressant medication, and women living with HIV/AIDS. Women who have a history of cervical cancer must continue to be screened with Pap smears indefinitely. In contrast, women who have undergone hysterectomy (with removal of the cervix) for reasons other than cervical dysplasia or cervical cancer do not need any further Pap smears postoperatively.

Pap smear screening can be stopped between the ages of 65 or 70, depending on the source of the guidelines: ACOG recommends cessation between 65 and 70, and the ASCCP/ACS/USPSTF draft guidelines recommend cessation of Pap testing by age 70. Termination of Pap smear screening also requires that women meet the exclusion criteria noted above—that at least 20 years have passed since a moderate or severe cervical dysplasia, and no significant immunosuppression. Importantly, while the peak incidence of cervical cancer among Caucasian women is in the 40s, it is in the 70s for Hispanic and Asian women, and increases throughout the lifespan for African American women. Therefore, it is important that prior history and screening be taken into account prior to discontinuing Pap smears (40).

Women often have some anxiety about stopping Pap smears, as they may fear that a cancer will be missed, or that their physicians are "abandoning" important screening practices simply because they are "too old." It is helpful to explain that the Pap smear screens only for cervical cancer, and that they will still have annual gynecologic exams to screen for ovarian cancer and other pathology.

7. HPV screening strategies

Screening tests for HPV have been available since 1999. Tests exist for both low risk and high risk HPV; however, since low risk HPV is not associated with carciongenesis, there are currently no clinical indications for low risk HPV testing. Some authors have even called for the low risk test to be removed from the market, as it does not appear to add any clinically useful information, and may contribute to confusion among clinicians about how and when to screen for HPV (44, 45). For high risk HPV subtypes, there are three currently available and FDA-approved tests; the best studied of these is Hybrid Capture, and further data are needed to assess the reliability of newer tests (46).

7.1 Reflex HPV testing for ASC-US Paps

Clinically, several strategies for using HPV tests have been employed. The first and most prevalent use of the HPV test is for the evaluation of a non-diagnostic Pap smear. Approximately 4% of Pap smears will result in a reading of "atypical squamous cells of undetermined significance," or ASC-US (47). These Paps may represent a wide spectrum of problems: non-specific inflammation, dysplasia of any severity, cervical cancer, or simply artifact. Further evaluation is therefore warranted; in 20-60% of women with an ASC-US Pap smear, dysplasia is present. The American Society for Colposcopy and Cervical Pathology (ASCCP) offers three management strategies: a repeat Pap smear in six months, an immediate colposcopic examination of the cervix, or HPV testing. If an HPV test is performed and is negative, the Pap is considered normal, and the woman can simply have a Pap in one year. If HPV testing is positive, then the suspicion for dysplasia is higher and colposcopy is recommended (48). Thus in the setting of ASC-US, a negative HPV test will reassure those women at low risk for dysplasia and allow them to avoid unnecessary procedures, and a positive HPV test will ensure that women at higher risk for dysplasia are rapidly evaluated. For clinicians using liquid-based cytology, the HPV test can be done on the same sample as the Pap smear, thus obviating the need for the patient to return for a second exam if ASC-US is found.

7.2 Automatic HPV testing

The other testing strategy is "automatic" HPV testing (rather than reflexively in response to the cytologic result), and is appropriate for women over the age of 30. It is important that women under 30 years of age not undergo routine or automatic HPV screening, as the prevalence of HPV among younger women is very high, and most of these infections are transient and without consequence. Among women over 30, however, transient HPV infections are less common, and the HPV test has a higher positive predictive value for cervical dysplasia (48).

When a woman over 30 has a cytologically normal Pap smear and a negative high risk HPV test, she is considered very low risk for cervical dysplasia and cancer, and should thereafter receive Pap smears *only every three years* (40, 48). Even if a woman acquires an HPV infection during that three year interval, the long incubation time between HPV acquisition and development of significant dysplasia means that her next Pap smear should still detect any new dysplasia in its early stages.

When a woman over 30 has a cytologically normal Pap smear and a positive high risk HPV test, current guidelines recommend repeating both tests in 12 months, as it is only *persistent* HPV infection that leads to dysplasia. If at 12 months the HPV test is persistently positive, or if a cytologic abnormality has developed in that interval, then colposcopy is recommended (48).

8. HPV vaccination

There are currently two commercially available prophylactic vaccines against HPV: a quadrivalent vaccine against strains 6, 11, 16, and 18, and a bivalent vaccine against 16 and 18. Neither vaccine has been studied long enough nor in a large enough number of women to demonstrate a reduction in cervical cancer among vaccines. However, both vaccines have demonstrated excellent immunogenicity against the targeted HPV strains, and have shown efficacy at reducing the surrogate endpoints of grade 2 and grade 3 cervical dysplasia (49-51). It is anticipated that high uptake of the vaccine will reduce the number of women requiring colposcopy and subsequent extirpative procedures, and ultimately reduce cervical cancer rates. However, several caveats must be added.

First, as vaccination protects against only two oncogenic strains, women remain vulnerable to other (non-vaccine) HPV strains, and therefore remain at some risk for cervical dysplasia and cancer. Both vaccines induce some cross-protection against non-vaccine strains, though this is far from perfect. Therefore, vaccinated women should continue to undergo Pap smears at the interval appropriate for their age and health status—the vaccine does not abrogate the need for Pap smears (40).

Second, availability and uptake of the vaccine has thus far been low for a variety of reasons. At present, approximately 37% of eligible girls in the United States have been vaccinated against HPV (52). There have been multiple barriers to its widespread adoption. These include parental uncertainty about the importance and timing of vaccinating young girls for a sexually transmitted disease, expense of the vaccine series, and even political posturing over the vaccine, to name a few. With widespread adoption, vaccination against HPV 16 and 18 has the potential to eliminate up to two thirds of cervical cancer worldwide (53). The highest burden of HPV disease and cervical cancer clearly lies in developing nations without easy access to cervical cancer screening. At present, the cost of the vaccine is such that it is not available to the populations most in need.

9. Barriers to adoption of evidence-based Pap smear screening

While the current Pap smear screening guidelines have been widely publicized and received considerable attention in the lay press when released, there remains ongoing evidence of Pap smear over-use by clinicians (44, 45, 54). There are a number of barriers to physician compliance with evidence-based treatment protocols. These include lack of awareness of the guidelines, lack of "buy-in" to the new recommendations, and inertia. In addition, patient expectations for an annual Pap smear may drive some Pap overuse, as it may be easier to accede to the patient's request than to spend limited visit time explaining HPV and the rationale for the new screening intervals. However, Pap smears performed too frequently or too early and HPV tests performed at inappropriate ages or intervals represent a significant cost to the health care system. Furthermore, there is the potential for patient harm when Pap smears are not performed according to current standards. For example, the diagnosis of HPV or a low grade dysplasia in an 18 year old woman may cause her real emotional distress, may result in her subjection to additional procedures such as colposcopies and biopsies, and possibly extirpative procedures. However, the 18 year old is likely to simply clear her HPV infection without intervention. By age 21, when her first Pap smear is due, one of two things will occur—she will have cleared her HPV, and her Pap smear will be normal, or she will have persistent dysplasia, in which case she merits further evaluation. The probability that she will have a cervical cancer is, as noted above, vanishingly small (41).

10. Areas of controversy and uncertainty

10.1 HPV triage: molecular screening for cervical cancer

As demonstrated in a large international study, the prevalence of HPV among documented cervical cancers was over 99%, which represents the largest attributable fraction ever identified for a cause of cancer (55). Therefore, significant interest exists in utilizing HPV testing as a primary screening modality. Several large clinical studies have been conducted to evaluate the efficacy of primary HPV screening and/or cotesting with conventional cytology. The Canadian Cervical Cancer Screening Trial evaluated the test characteristics of HPV testing with conventional cytology in 10, 154 women aged 30-69 who underwent both tests. Consistent with prior studies, the sensitivity of HPV testing for the detection of CIN 2 or greater was significantly higher than that of conventional cytology (96.4% versus 55.4%) and the specificity was lower (94.1% versus 96.8%) (27, 56, 57).

A population-based screening study in Amsterdam randomly assigned approximately 17,000 women to either cytology/HPV co-testing or cytology alone at an initial screen. These women were then followed with cytology/HPV co-testing at 5 years (the standard screening interval in the Netherlands). Results of CIN 3 or worse were detected in 70% more women in the group undergoing cytology/HPV co-testing at initial screening, and women in this group were less likely to have CIN3 or worse detected at the five year follow-up screening test. Overall, the number of cases of CIN3 lesions or cancers did not differ between trial arms, suggesting that initial co-testing may detect significant lesions earlier but not any more effectively than conventional cytologic screening (58). Similar results were obtained in a large study conducted in England (59).

A recent randomized controlled trial from Italy that evaluated conventional cytology compared with HPV DNA testing in over 47,000 women provides additional information regarding the efficacy of HPV screening as a primary modality (60). In this study, initial screening with HPV DNA testing reduced the number of invasive cervical cancers discovered at a second round of screening (0 cases with HPV screening, 9 cases with conventional cytology). Additionally, women screened with HPV testing were noted to have an excess number of cases of CIN 2 or greater over the two rounds of screening. Therefore, this study represents the first evidence that primary screening with HPV testing decreases the incidence of cervical cancer with earlier detection. However, HPV testing also leads to the overdiagnosis of women with CIN 2 or worse lesions that would have spontaneously regressed without treatment.

Lastly, a long-term prospective cohort study of over 330,000 women in a Northern California health-maintenance organization has provided interesting new data on the safety and efficacy of cytology/HPV cotesting. This study demonstrated that patients with an initial negative HPV test demonstrated an extremely low risk of CIN3 or worse over the subsequent 5 years. The risk was practically equal for those with negative and ASCUS cytologies and a negative initial HPV test. Notably, the cumulative 5-year risk of cancer was lower in those with negative HPV tests compared with negative cytology at the initial screen (3.8 per 100,000 compared with 7.5 per 100,000). The authors concluded that a single negative HPV test is sufficiently reassuring against a 5-year risk of cancer. They also advocated for a triage strategy of primary HPV testing with positive results undergoing triage by cytology (54).

While findings from these (and many other) studies vary in magnitude, consistent observations are noteworthy. Compared with cytology, HPV testing offers a highly reproducible, objective outcome that is easily monitored. Compared with cytology alone, HPV testing is more sensitive, less specific, and has a higher negative predictive value (27, 56, 57). The lower sensitivity relative to conventional cytology is significant in that with primary HPV screening, significantly more women would be recommended for unnecessary colposcopies for transient HPV infections, which would consume substantial health care resources. This phenomenon is particularly true for women under age 30, who have the highest incidence of HPV infection and the lowest rates of cervical cancer. The addition of HPV testing to conventional cytology may result in the earlier diagnosis of high grade lesions or cancer and may reduce the incidence of caner (evidence from one clinical trial), however a mortality benefit has not been demonstrated to date. Thus, additional study regarding the optimal screening strategy is required.

10.2 Visual inspection with acetic acid and "Screen and Treat" programs

Historically, visual inspection of the cervix without magnification was the initial screening test for cervical cancer. Introduced by Schiller in the 1930s, the test was initially performed by applying Lugol's iodine to the cervix (61). The test was rapidly replaced by Pap testing, which demonstrated improved specificity. However, visual inspection of the cervix, after the application of either acetic acid or Lugol's solution, remains a mainstay of cervical cancer screening in resource-poor settings given that the technique requires little equipment, provides rapid results, and is economical.

A substantial body of literature exists supporting the efficacy of visual inspection techniques and "screen and treat" protocols. Regarding test characteristics, observational studies have evaluated the sensitivity and specificity of visual inspection, which were noted to be 79% and 85% respectively in a meta-analysis of 11 of the higher quality studies (62). The efficacy of visual inspection as a part of "screen and treat" programs has also been evaluated in a number of studies. A large randomized controlled trial in India that evaluated over 80,000 women assigned to either triage with visual inspection followed by cryotherapy or excision versus standard therapy (health education). The visual inspection protocol decreased cervical cancer incidence and mortality (63). Additionally, a large randomized trial from South Africa evaluated the efficacy of two distinct screen and treat protocols in 6500 previously unscreened women. All women in the trial were screened with visual inspection, HPV testing, and cytology and were then randomized to one of three treatment arms: cryotherapy for positive HPV test, cryotherapy for positive visual inspection, or delayed evaluation (follow-up at 6 months). At the 6 and 12 month follow-up colposcopic evaluations, significantly fewer women were noted to have CIN 2 or worse in the HPV and visual inspections groups compared with conventional cytology (64).

Therefore, while conventional screening programs remain the backbone of cervical cancer prevention, visual inspection and screen and treat protocols provide options for women in low-resource settings where screening programs remain unavailable. These protocols provide opportunities for efficient, safe, and effective treatment of women and eliminate any potential problems related to communication barriers and non-compliance with follow-up. Additional research and resources must be directed toward the evaluation and implementation of effective screening and treatment protocols in low-resource settings.

10.3 Conventional Pap screening versus liquid-based cytology

With "conventional" Pap screening, cells obtained from the cervix are transferred directly to a glass slide with fixation by either ethyl alcohol or other spray fixative. Liquid-based cytology refers to the technology whereby cervical cells are suspended in a liquid transport medium and then displayed on a glass slide in the laboratory. Liquid-based cytology improves specimen adequacy by minimizing artifact, such as inflammation, non-cellular debris, and epithelial cell clumping, which may obscure interpretation of the smear. However, while the uniform cell layer from liquid-based cytology allows for easier interpretation, pathologists and cytotechnologists cannot use the additional information provided by background inflammation as clues facilitating diagnosis. In addition, large systematic review challenged the clinical relevance of this difference in adequacy by failing to discover a difference in the number of unsatisfactory slides (65). One significant advantage conferred by liquid-based cytology is the ability to collect reflex HPV testing, which otherwise must be obtained by a separate sample in systems using conventional cytology.

At the time liquid-based cytology was developed, the test was marketed as a more sensitive screening test than conventional cytology which was supported by early studies with clear methodological inadequacies (66-69). Recent studies have challenged this notion, and to date, the question remains largely unanswered (20, 70, 71). A systematic review of 56 published studies that included over 1 million slides recently addressed the current literature on this subject (19). Regarding study design, no studies were noted to be "ideal" but five were considered to be of high-quality. The authors concluded that liquid-based cytology offered no improvement over conventional cytology for the detection of high-grade lesions. Other systematic and independent reviews have reported similar findings (18, 72). Observational data suggest that liquid-based samples may improve the detection of glandular lesions (73-75).

Arguably, the liquid-based Pap screening test is not a "better" test than conventional cytology. However, despite the increased cost, the liquid-based screen offers advantages that will maintain its use in developed countries, particularly the United States. In the 2006 screening guidelines, the American Society for Colposcopy and Cervical Pathology endorses reflex HPV testing as the preferred triage strategy for an ASCUS Pap result, which is supported by data from a large, well-designed clinical trial (37, 76). Therefore, given the ease of HPV testing with liquid-based samples and the current available infrastructure, the return of conventional cytology to the US is unlikely. However, should primary HPV screening with reflex cytology for positive results be adopted in the future, liquid based screening may become a less cost effective strategy given that the number of samples will decline. Importantly, the aforementioned studies support the use of conventional cytology as a safe, effective, and cost-effective screening strategy in settings with limited resources.

11. Conclusions

- The Pap smear is the single most successful cancer screening tool in modern medicine.
- Cervical cancer is due to persistent infection with high-risk, oncogenic HPV strains.
- Even in women with documented high-grade dysplasia (CIN 2 or greater), a long premalignant window exists which allows for purposeful intervention and prevention of progression to malignancy.
- As a result, newer screening recommendations have decreased screening intervals to maximize the benefit of screening and decrease unnecessary interventions
- As our understanding of HPV increases, Pap smear screening intervals continue to decline and triage strategies may change. It is imperative that practitioners remain informed of evidence-based guidelines.
- Despite the availability of screening and preventative strategies, the majority of the cervical cancer disease burden is in the developing world. Inequalities in the availability of screening are a substantial public health challenge.

- Universal vaccination against HPV has the potential to substantially reduce the cervical cancer disease burden worldwide, however cost and other barrier currently limited the widespread adoption of this strategy.

12. References

[1] Papanicolaou GN, Traut HF. The diagnostic value of vaginal smears in carcinoma of the uterus. Am J Obstet Gynecol. 1941;42:193-206.

[2] Ries L, Eisner MP, Kosary CL, et al.SEER Cancer Statistics Review, 1975–2002. Bethesda, MD: National Cancer Institute, 2004.

[3] Jemal A, Siegel R, Ward E et al. Cancer statistics, 2006. CA Cancer J Clin 2006;56:106–130

[4] U.S. Department of Health and Human Services.Healthy People 2010. Washington, DC: U.S. Government Printing Office, 2000.

[5] Sawaya GF, Grimes DA. New technologies in cervical cytology screening: a word of caution, Obstetrics & Gynecology 94(2), August 1999, p 307–310.

[6] Pund ER, Nieburgs H, Nettles JB, et al. Preinvasive carcinoma of the cervix uteri: seven cases in which it was detected by examination of routine endocervical smears. Arch Pathol Lab Med 1947;44: 571–577.

[7] Meisels A, Fortin R, Roy M. Condylomatous lesions of the cervix. II. Cytologic, colposcopic and histopathologic study. Acta Cytol 1977;21:379–390.

[8] Beckmann AM, Myerson D, Daling JR, et al. Detection and localization of human papillomavirus DNA in human genital condylomas by in situ hybridization with biotinylated probes. J Med Virol 1985;16:265–273.

[9] zur Hausen, H. Condylomata acuminata and human genital cancer. Cancer Res. 36, 530, 1976.

[10] M. Dürst, L. Gissmann, H. Ikenberg, and H. zur Hausen: A papillomavirus DNA from a cervical carcinoma and its prevalence in cancer biopsy samples from different geographic regions. Proc. Nat. Acad. Sci. U.S. 80, 3812-3815, 1983.

[11] M. Boshart, L. Gissmann, H. Ikenberg, A. Kleinheinz, W. Scheurlen, and H. zur Hausen: A new type of papillomavirus DNA, its presence in genital cancer and in cell lines derived from genital cancer. EMBO J. 3, 1151-1157,1984.

[12] Katz, DL. Fundamentals of screening: the art and science of looking for trouble. In: Clinical epidemiology and evidence based medicine - fundamental principals of evidence based medicine and research. Sage Publications, London 2001. p69-90.

[13] Fletcher RH, Fletcher SW. Prevention. In: Clinical epidemiology - The Essentials, 4th ed. Lippincott Williams & Wilkins, Baltimore 2005. p147-167.

[14] Mandel JS, Bond JH, and Church TR et al. Reducing mortality from colorectal cancer by screening for fecal occult blood. Minnesota Colon Cancer Control Study. N Engl J Med. 1993;328:1365.

[15] Welch HG. Screening mammography—a long run for a short slide? N Engl J Med. 2010; 363(13): 1276-7.

[16] Nanda K, McCrory DC, Myers ER, Bastian LA, Hasselblad V, Hickey JD, Matchar DB. Accuracy of the Papanicolaou test in screening for and follow-up of cervical

cytologic abnormalities: a systematic review. Ann Intern Med. 2000 May 16;132(10):810-9.
[17] Mayrand MH, Duarte-Franco E, Rodrigues I, Walter SD, Hanley J, Ferenczy A, Ratnam S, Coutlée F, Franco EL; Canadian Cervical Cancer Screening Trial Study Group. Human papillomavirus DNA versus Papanicolaou screening tests for cervical cancer. N Engl J Med. 2007 Oct 18;357(16):1579-88.
[18] Arbyn M., Bergeron C., Klinkhamer P., et al: Liquid compared with conventional cervical cytology: a systematic review and meta-analysis. *Obstet Gynecol* 2008; 111:167-77.
[19] Davey E., Barratt A., Irwig L.: Effect of study design and quality on unsatisfactory rates, cytology classifications, and accuracy in liquid-based versus conventional cervical cytology: a systematic review. *Lance. 2006;* 367:122-32.
[20] Ronco G., Cuzick J., Pierotti P., et al: Accuracy of liquid based versus conventional cytology: overall results of new technologies for cervical cancer screening: randomised controlled trial. *BMJ*. 2007; 335: 28.
[21] Vilos GA. Dr. George Papanicolaou and the birth of the pap test. Obstet Gynecol Surv. 1999; 54:481-83.
[22] Papanicolaou GN. New cancer diagnosis. In: Proceedings of the Third Race Betterment Conference, 1928. 2-5 Jan: Battle Creek, MI: pp528-34.
[23] American Cancer Society. Guidelines for the cancer related checkup: recommendations and rationale. CA Cancer J Clin. 1980;30:195-230.
[24] Burns EL, Hammond EC, Percy C, et al. Detection of uterine cancer. Results of a community program of 17 years. Cancer. 1968;22:1108-1119.
[25] Hammond EC, Seidman H. Progress in control of cancer of the uterus. Arch Environ Health. 1966;13:105-116.
[26] Christopherson WM, Mendez WM, Ahuja EM, et al. Cervix cancer control in Louisville, Kentucky. Cancer. 1970;26:29-38.
[27] Waxman AG. Guidelines for cervical cancer screening: history and scientific rationale. Clin Obstet Gynecol. 2005; 48(1): 77-97.
[28] Gustafsson L, Ponten J, Bergstrom R & Adami HO. International incidence rates of invasive cervical cancer before cytological screening. International Journal of Cancer 1997; 71: 159–165
[29] U.S. Cancer Statistics Working Group. United States Cancer Statistics: 1999–2007 Incidence and Mortality Web-based Report. Atlanta (GA): Department of Health and Human Services, Centers for Disease Control and Prevention, and National Cancer Institute; 2010. Available at: http://www.cdc.gov/uscs.
[30] Howlader N, Noone AM, Krapcho M, Neyman N, Aminou R, Waldron W, Altekruse SF, Kosary CL, Ruhl J, Tatalovich Z, Cho H, Mariotto A, Eisner MP, Lewis DR, Chen HS, Feuer EJ, Cronin KA, Edwards BK (eds). *SEER Cancer Statistics Review, 1975-2008*, National Cancer Institute. Bethesda, MD, http://seer.cancer.gov/csr/1975_2008/, based on November 2010 SEER data submission, posted to the SEER web site, 2011.
[31] Sankaranarayanan R, Ferlay J. Worldwide burden of gyaecological cancer: the size of the problem. Best Pract Res Clinc Obstet Gynaecol. 2006;20:207-225.

[32] World Health Organization. Strengthening cervical cancer prevention and control. Report of the GAVI-UNFPA-WHO meeting. December 2009. Geneva, Switzerland.
[33] Berek and Novak's Gynecology. pp 562-571. Ed: Berek, J. Lippincott Williams and Wilkins: Philadelphia, 2007.
[34] Einstein MH, Schiller JT, Viscidi RP, Strickler HD, Coursaget P, Tan T, Halsey N and Jenkins D. Clinician's guide to human papillomavirus immunology: knowns and unknowns. The Lancet Infectious Diseases, 9(6), June 2009, pp 347-356.
[35] Tjalma WAA, Van Waes TR, Van den Eeden LEM, and Bogers JJPM. Role of human papillomavirus in the carcinogenesis of squamous cell carcinoma and adenocarcinoma of the cervix. Best Practice & Research Clinical Obstetrics & Gynaecology, 19(4) August 2005, pp 469-483.
[36] Ho GY, Bierman R, Beardsley L, et al. Natural history of cervicovaginal papillomavirus infection in young women. N Engl J Med 1998; 338:423- 428.
[37] Wright TC, Massad LS, Dunton CJ, Spitzer M, Wilkinson EJ, Solomon D for the 2006 American Society for Colposcopy and Cervical Pathology–sponsored Consensus Conference. 2006 consensus guidelines for the management of women with abnormal cervical cancer screening tests. AJOG 2007, 197(4), pp 346-355.
[38] Atkins KA, Jeronimo J, Stoler MH. ALTS Group. Description of patients with squamous cell carcinoma in the atypical squamous cells of undetermined significance/low-grade squamous intraepithelial lesion triage study. Cancer. 108(4): 212-21, 2006 Aug 25.
[39] Moscicki AB, Schiffman M, Kjaer S, Villa LL. Chapter 5: updating the natural history of HPV and anogenital cancer. Vaccine 2006; 24(S3): 42–51.
[40] ACOG Practice Bulletin 109: Cervical Cytology Screening. Obstet Gynecol 2009; 114 (6): 1409-1420.
[41] Watson M, Saraiya M, Benard V, Coughlin SS, Flowers L, Cokkinides V, et al. Burden of cervical cancer in the United States, 1998-2003. Cancer 2008; 113(suppl): 2855–64.
[42] ASCCP draft consensus guidelines: http://www.asccp.org/PracticeManagement/PICSM/TheRoleofMolecularTesting Symposium/tabid/9856/Default.aspx (accessed 10/25/11).
[43] Whitlock EP, Vesco KK, Eder M, Lin JS, Senger CA, Burda BU. Liquid-Based Cytology and Human Papillomavirus Testing to Screen for Cervical Cancer: A Systematic Review for the U.S. Preventive Services Task Force. Ann Int Med 2011 (Epub ahead of print).
[44] Lee JW, Berkowitz Z, Saraiya M. Low-Risk Human Papillomavirus Testing and Other Nonrecommended Human Papillomavirus Testing Practices Among U.S. Health Care Providers. Obstet Gynecol 2011; 118: 4–13.
[45] Saraiya M, Berkowitz Z, Yabroff KR, Wideroff L, Kobrin S, Benard V. Cervical cancer screening with both human papillomavirus and Papanicolaou testing vs Papanicolaou testing alone: what screening intervals are physicians recommending? Arch Intern Med 2010; 170: 977–85.
[46] Kinney W, Stoler MH, Castle PE. Special commentary: patient safety and the next generation of HPV DNA tests. Am J Clin Pathol. 2010; 134: 193-9.

[47] Solomon D, Schiffman M, Tarone R for the ALTS Group. Comparison of Three Management Strategies for Patients With Atypical Squamous Cells of Undetermined Significance: Baseline Results From a Randomized Trial. J Natl Cancer Inst (2001) 93 (4): 293-299.

[48] Wright TC, Massad LS, Dunton CJ, Spitzer M, Wilkinson EJ, Solomon D, for the 2006 American Society for Colposcopy and Cervical Pathology–sponsored Consensus Conference. 2006 consensus guidelines for the management of women with abnormal cervical cancer screening tests. 2007; 197(4): 346-355.

[49] The FUTURE II Study Group. Quadrivalent vaccine against human papillomavirus to prevent high-grade cervical lesions. N Engl J Med. 2007; 356(19): 1915–1927.

[50] Villa, LL et al. Prophylactic quadrivalent human papillomavirus (types 6, 11, 16, and 18) L1 virus-like particle vaccine in young women: a randomised double-blind placebo-controlled multicentre phase II efficacy trial. Lancet Oncology 2005 6(5): 271-279.

[51] Einstein MH et al on behalf of the HPV-010 study group. Comparison of the immunogenicity and safety of CervarixTM and Gardasil ® human papillomavirus (HPV) cervical cancer vaccines in healthy women aged 18–45 years. Human Vaccines 5(10), 705-719; October 2009.

[52] Centers for Disease Control and Prevention (CDC). National, state, and local area vaccination coverage among adolescents aged 13–17 years—United States, 2008. MMWR Morb Mortal Wkly Rep 2009; 58:997–1001.

[53] Smith JS, Lindsay L, Hoots B, Keys J, Franceschi S, Winer R. and Clifford GM. Human papillomavirus type distribution in invasive cervical cancer and high-grade cervical lesions: A meta-analysis update. International Journal of Cancer, 2007; 121: 621–632.

[54] Katki HA, Kinney WK, Fetterman B, et al. Cervical cancer risk for women undergoing concurrent testing for human papillomavirus and cervical cytology: a population-based study in routine clinical practice. Lancet Oncol. 2011; 12:663-72.

[55] Walboomers JM, Jacobs MV, Manos MM, et al. Human papillomavirus is a necessary cause of invasive cervical cancer worldwide. J Pathol 1999;189:12-9.

[56] Mayrand MH, Duarte-Franco E, Mansour N, et al. Human Papillomavirus DNA versus Papanicolaou screening tests for cervical cancer. N Engl N Med 2007; 357: 1579-88

[57] Koliopolous G, Arbyn M, Martin-Hirsch P, et al. Diagnostiuc accuracy of human papillomavirus testing in primary cervical screening: a systematic review and meta-analysis of non-randomized trials. Gynecol Oncol 2007;104:232-46.

[58] Bulkmans NW, Berkhof J, Rozendaal L et al. Human papillomavirus DNA testing for the detection of cervical intraepithelial neoplasia grade 3 and cancer: 5-year follow-up of a randomised controlled implementation trial. Lancet. 2007;370(9601):1764.

[59] Kitchener HC, Almonte M, Thomson C, et al. HPV testing in combination with liquid-based cytology in primary cervical screening (ARTISTIC): a randomised controlled trial. Lancet Oncol. 2009;10(7):672.

[60] Ronco G, Giorgi-Rossi P, Carozzi F, et al. New Technologies for Cervical Cancer screening (NTCC) Working Group. Efficacy of human papillomavirus testing for

the detection of invasive cervical cancers and cervical intraepithelial neoplasia: a randomised controlled trial. Lancet Oncol. 2010;11(3):249.

[61] Schiller, W. Leucoplakia, leucokeratosis, and carcinoma of the cervix. Am J Obstet Gynecol 1938; 35:17

[62] Arbyn M, Sankaranarayanan R, Muwonge R, et al. Pooled analysis of the accuracy of five cervical cancer screening tests assessed in eleven studies in Africa and India. Int J Cancer. 2008;123(1):153

[63] Sankaranarayanan R, Esmy PO, Rajkumar R, Muwonge R, et al. Effect of visual screening on cervical cancer incidence and mortality in Tamil Nadu, India: a cluster-randomised trial. Lancet. 2007;370(9585):398

[64] Denny L, Kuhn L, De Souza M, Pollack AE, Dupree W, Wright TC. Screen-and-treat approaches for cervical cancer prevention in low-resource settings: a randomized controlled trial. JAMA. 2005;294(17):2173

[65] Davey E, Barratt A, Irwig L, Chan SF, Macaskill P, Mannes P, Saville AM. Effect of study design and quality on unsatisfactory rates, cytology classifications, and accuracy in liquid-based versus conventional cervical cytology: a systematic review. Lancet. 2006;367(9505):122.

[66] Diaz-Rosario I.A., Kabawai S.E.: Performance of a fluid-based, thin-layer Papanicolaou smear method in the clinical setting of an independent laboratory and an outpatient screening population in New England. *Arch Pathol Lab Med.* 1999;123:817-21.

[67] Carpenter A.B., Davey D.D.: ThinPrep Pap test: performance and biopsy follow-up in a university hospital. *Cancer.* 1999;87:105-12.

[68] Papillo J.L., Zarka M.A., St John T.L.: Evaluation of the ThinPrep Pap test in clinical practice. A seven-month, 16,314-case experience in northern Vermont. *Acta Cytol.* 1998; 42:203-8.

[69] Hutchinson M.L., Zahniser D.J., Shrman M.F., et al: Utility of liquid-based cytology for cervical carcinoma screening: results of a population-based study conducted in a region of Costa Rica with a high incidence of cervical carcinoma. *Cancer.* 1999;87:48-55.

[70] Coste J., Cochand-Priollet B., de Cremoux P., et al: Cross-sectional study of conventional cervical smear, monolayer cytology, and human papillomavirus DNA testing for cervical cancer screening. *BMJ.* 2003;326:733-7.

[71] Taylor S., Kuhn L., Dupree W., et al: Direct comparison of liquid-based and conventional cytology in a South African screening trial. *Int J Cancer.* 2006;118:957-62.

[72] Abulafia O, Pezzullo JC, Sherer DM. Performance of ThinPrep liquid-based cervical cytology in comparison with conventionally prepared Papanicolaou smears: a quantitative survey. Gynecol Oncol. 2003;90(1):137.

[73] Hecht JL, Sheets EE, Lee KR. Atypical glandular cells of undetermined significance in conventional cervical/vaginal smears and thin-layer preparations. Cancer. 2002;96(1):1.

[74] Lee KR, Darragh TM, Joste NE, Krane JF, Sherman ME, Hurley LB, Allred EM, Manos MM. Atypical glandular cells of undetermined significance (AGUS): Interobserver

reproducibility in cervical smears and corresponding thin-layer preparations. Am J Clin Pathol. 2002;117(1):96.
[75] Wang N, Emancipator SN, Rose P, Rodriguez M, Abdul-Karim FW. Histologic follow-up of atypical endocervical cells. Liquid-based, thin-layer preparation vs. conventional Pap smear. Acta Cytol. 2002;46(3):453.
[76] Results of a randomized trial on the management of cytology interpretations of atypical squamous cells of undetermined significance. The ASCUS-LSIL Triage Study (ALTS) Group. *Am J Obstet Gynecol*. 2003;188;1383-92.

9

Evidence-Based Medicine – Perspectives of a Community-Based Pediatrician

Richard Haber
Pediatric Consultation Center,
Montreal Children's Hospital,
McGill University
Canada

1. Introduction

Have we succumbed to a new tyranny in medicine—evidence-based medicine? With apologies to my former professor, Dr. David Sackett! but has the randomized controlled trial (RCT) become a new idol? Indeed, EBM has been satirized as a new religion.[1] At the risk of not being 'politically correct",[2] I would argue that evidence-based medicine (EBM) can be abused and substituted for sound clinical judgment. The exponents of the new paradigm we call evidence-based medicine recognized this: "Thus, knowing the tools of evidence-based practice is necessary but not sufficient for delivering the highest quality of patient care. In addition to clinical expertise, the clinician requires compassion, sensitive listening skills, and broad perspectives from the humanities and social sciences."[3] Evidence-based medicine, when properly understood and applied, improves patient outcomes but it is often misunderstood and used inappropriately.[4] It is important to recognize the limitations of EBM as well as its benefits in the care of our patients. Strauss and McAlister point out some of the limitations of EBM[5]: " shortage of coherent, consistent scientific evidence, difficulties in applying evidence to the care of individual patients, barriers to the practice of high-quality medicine, limited time and resources, paucity of evidence that evidence-based medicine works." One common example that many community generalists would share around the concept of 'barriers to the practice of high-quality medicine' is the issue of a lack of resources for the appropriate care of one's patient. For example, there is an unacceptable waiting time for a child you suspect of having autism to see a child psychiatrist to confirm the diagnosis and enable the family to obtain publicly funded resources for early intervention. This is equally true for other psychiatric disorders. Indeed, the wait time for many subspecialties in pediatrics is often in the order of many months.

Evidence-based medicine is an offshoot of the philosophical movement known as scientific positivism. Scientific positivism is a particular philosophy, which states that only that which is scientifically verifiable is true. The critique of scientific positivism is that its central premise is itself not scientifically verifiable but must be accepted as a sort of first principle or axiom. Similarly, the principle of evidence-based medicine must be itself accepted as an axiom of the system. This can be seen if we frame the following question, 'what is the evidence that evidence-based medicine improves patient outcomes?' In fact, there is no such evidence since such a trial would be extremely difficult and unethical to do. "Evidence-based medicine, like other models of care, has limitations ...efforts need to be directed toward ... conducting studies to test whether and how evidence-based medicine affects processes of care and patient outcomes."[6]

Let me clearly state that my comments are not to be taken as an excuse to return to magical thinking or charlatanism. The outstanding achievements of modern medicine have been accomplished through the rigorous application of the scientific method in developing evidence-based guidelines. Patient outcomes have certainly improved with the application of these treatments. We are also aware of therapeutic disasters when the principles of controlled observations and rigorous research designs are not observed. (eg tying off the internal mammary arteries in the treatment for angina pectoris[7]).

Having said this, there is an *a priori* reason why we should not substitute evidence-based medicine for a more holistic approach and that is quite simply that the evidence is never complete. This is a fundamental feature of the scientific method and it is applicable in all the sciences. Recently, for example, the most fundamental aspect of Einstein's theory of special relativity, the fixed speed of light (299,792,458 m/sec) has been challenged by experiments at OPERA which demonstrated that neutrinos travel slightly faster than the speed of light.[8] If this finding is duplicated by other laboratories, then our understanding of the fundamental features of space-time will need to be revised. Until this announcement, it was unthinkable that Einstein's constant was not true since his theory of special relativity made many predictions subsequently validated by observation. However, this latest challenge to Einstein should not surprise us because the basic hermeneutic underlying the scientific method depends on theories *validated by observations;* as the observations change through more and more sophisticated technological advances, the theories need to be modified. Physicists have yet to achieve the unifying theory which combines Einstein's theory of special relativity and quantum mechanics which at present are incompatible. Evidence-based medicine is based on the scientific method and it is subject to the same caveats as physics and cosmology. Theoretically, the evidence base will continue to unfold *ad infinitum* since there is no principle which enables us to know that the end of the evidence has been reached and there can be no further evidence. We can only act in the concrete world of sick patients with the evidence at hand, as best as it, knowing that perhaps further evidence will prove us wrong.

A recent discussion in the New England Journal of Medicine highlights this problem and introduces a new dynamic.[9] The authors relate the case of a 13 year-old girl with lupus erythematosus with nephritic syndrome, antiphospholipid antibodies and pancreatitis. They site the difficulty of knowing whether or not to anticoagulate this patient since there is no data in the pediatric literature on this question. There would also be the danger of inducing bleeding. A survey of other pediatric rheumatologists did not produce a consensus. Since there were no RCT's on this question, the authors state that they turned to their hospital's EMR database and within the space of a few hours obtained their experience over the previous five years to arrive at an 'electronic cohort'. Through this retrospective analysis they opted to treat their patient with anticoagulants. This was not a RCT of anticoagulants versus no anticoagulants in a selected group of patients with SLE but physicians using their judgment based on past experience. "Did we make the correct decision for our patient? Thrombosis did not develop, and the patient did not have any sequelae related to her anticoagulation; truthfully, though, we may never really know. We will, however, know that we made the decision on the basis of the best data available—acting...in the light of experience guided by intelligence."[10]

There is always the possibility of newer evidence that will invalidate a particular diagnosis, therapeutic choice or diagnostic test. Newer diagnostic tools inevitably result in a greater understanding of pathophysiology, e.g. the explosion of molecular genetics. Often, there is no definitive RCT in the literature to help one with a clinical decision. Sometimes the results of a Cochrane summary, i.e the evaluation of available RCT's regarding a particular question, are contradictory or inconclusive.[11] One could also argue that the 'gold standard' RCT is best used when a clearly defined therapy is being tested i.e. drug A vs drug B in a well-defined group of patients. This may be the case in a secondary or tertiary care center but is not the case in primary care where multiple pathologies may be at work in a broader group of patients. An RCT may not be the most useful tool when evaluating problems in primary care where there is a less highly selected group of patients with a single defined etiology. [12] The outcome measure used in an RCT may be inappropriate as in the case of rosiglitazone where the primary outcome measure was the lowering of glycated hemoglobin. The clinical trials leading up to the release of this drug on the markets focused on an outcome that may not be relevant (glycemic control) and ignored important side effects, assuming that a reduction in glycated hemoglobin translates into improved patient outcome. Indeed the side effects (weight gain, edema, and changes in lipids) detected during the clinical trials may well be more important with regard to outcome than glycemic control. Nissen and Wolski in fact showed that rosiglitazone increases the risks of myocardial infarction, despite improved glycemic control. [13]

Recently, Ioannidis has argued cogently that much published research is eventually shown to be false. This results from the attempts to achieve a conclusive result based on a single study assessed statistically using a p value of <.05. "A finding from a well-conducted, adequately powered randomized controlled trial starting with a 50% pre-study chance that the intervention is effective is eventually true about 85% of the time. ...Conversely, a meta-analytic finding from inconclusive studies where pooling is used to "correct" the low power of single studies, is probably false if R=<1:3. Research findings from underpowered, early-phase clinical trials would be true about one in four times, or even less frequently if bias is present."[14] There is also a darker side to the quest for evidence-based guidelines when vital evidence is withheld from the public domain, or falsified, invalidating the 'evidence' upon which a particular therapy is recommended. An example of this occurred with the clinical trials of a new iron-chelator, deferiprone. Apotex, the pharmaceutical firm developing the new drug, would not allow the publication of negative data. While researching a new iron-chelating agent, deferiprone, for Apotex, Nancy Olivieri of the Hospital for Sick Children in Toronto, uncovered data indicating that the drug would not provide long-term control of iron overload in patients with thalassemia major and worsened hepatic fibrosis. The pharmaceutical firm funding her research, Apotex, would not allow her to publish the data because of a research contract. Dr. Olivieri published the data regardless [15]and a major controversy regarding academic freedom ensued at great personal cost to Dr. Olivieri.[16] Another example is that of the COX-2 inhibitors. In the enthusiasm to release a new drug, rofecoxib, a COX-2 inhibitor, Bombardier et al[17] overlooked an important cardiovascular side effect in a subgroup of patients even though the drug showed promise in the group of patients for which the clinical trial was designed, those with rheumatoid arthritis. Subsequent analysis of the data indicating a substantial risk for cardiovascular events in patients taking the drug, resulted in the withdrawal of rofecoxib(Vioxx) from the market. . This has recently led to the institution of a registry for all RCT's; any researcher who wishes to publish in any of the major medical journals will now have to insure that their RCT is registered in the public domain, with all data both positive and negative available.[18]

There is also the moral issue of using data from trials conducted unethically as in the infamous Tuskegee Syphilis study in which 399 poor black sharecroppers were denied effective treatment so that researchers could follow the natural history of syphilis.[19]Similar comments can be made about the Nazi doctors and the use of eponyms such as Hallervorden-Spatz syndrome, honouring a pathologist, Hallervorden, who actively participated in the Nazi euthanasia program in order to obtain specimens of human brains for his research.[20]

Evidence can be published in recognized medical journals that is false because it has been unethically manipulated to justify a particular conclusion. Such was the case of the unjustified link between MMR immunization and autism published in The Lancet by Dr. Andrew Wakefield.[21] This publication was not only wrong but the data was manipulated as was shown by Brian Deer's exposé published in the British Medical Journal in 2011.[22] Wakefield postulated that 12 children had a 'new syndrome' of enterocolitis and regressive autism. In fact, 3/12 patients did not have regressive autism. 5/12 had a previous diagnosis of developmental problems long before receiving MMR vaccine and the symptoms of autism occurred months after the MMR was given and not within days. The study was further biased by the fact that the patients were recruited by known anti-MMR campaigners. Furthermore Dr. Wakefield stood to make financial gain through litigation by suing the pharmaceutical firms manufacturing the vaccine if his 'research' was generally accepted. The Lancet subsequently retracted the article in 2010 after untold damage had been done.[23] The false link between MMR and autism has caused needless worry to parents and along with other factors has led to a decline in herd immunity to measles with resultant increase in the number of cases in the developed world, where previously measles had almost been eliminated. As of October 2011, 26,074 cases of measles have been reported in European member states, with 14,000 cases in France alone. This has resulted in 7288 hospitalizations and 9 deaths.[24] Thus, while evidence-based practice is desirable, it is not always possible because of contamination of the evidence by either incomplete or changing evidence, and unethical manipulation of evidence. Because of these failures, evidence-based medicine cannot always lead to the healing and relief from suffering that our patients seek. Paradoxically, they turn to complementary and alternative medicine (CAM) which often has less of an evidence base than traditional medicine.

A further issue is that conclusions drawn from RCT's are based on a statistical assessment of the participants in the clinical trial but you must apply the conclusion to your particular patient. The danger is that your particular patient may not be similar to the patients in the clinical trial. This is especially a problem when trying to apply the results of a study, which has been done in a secondary or tertiary care center. The patients enrolled in such a trial may be quite different than the patients seen in a community practice. At any given clinical encounter, the physician does not have all the information needed to make an evidence-based decision. For example, every individual patient has a particular pharmacogenetic profile, which is largely unknown. Another major problem in pediatrics is, of course, that most drugs are 'orphans' i.e. there is no good information derived from studies in pediatrics and so we 'extrapolate' from adult studies. It is good to remind oneself that 'extrapolation' means that we are outside the principle of evidence-based medicine—we are extrapolating or going beyond the evidence on an assumption. The assumption is that what holds true for adult patients will hold true for pediatric patients. Of course, the 'assumption' is not evidence-based! Moreover, we now know that this assumption is often untrue. Consequently, evidence-based principles sometimes 'break down' in the concrete world in which individual physicians must act.

The renowned mediaeval philosopher/theologian Thomas Aquinas made a distinction, derived from Aristotle, between the speculative and practical intellect. The speculative intellect is the locus of analytical, theoretical thinking and this is the home of evidence-based medicine. The practical intellect, however, is the locus of applying evidence-based medicine to the practice of medicine: the specific judgment (having taken into account the evidence and the particulars of this patient before me) that the physician makes in determining the appropriateness of a particular treatment. The practical intellect is the final common pathway leading to a particular judgment for a particular patient. Let us take an example. A 9 year old girl is brought to your office at 5:00 PM on a Friday afternoon complaining of an earache. You correctly diagnose an otitis media. Evidence-based medicine would suggest that the correct course is not to prescribe an antibiotic but rather to prescribe analgesics and re-examine the patient 48 hours later; if no resolution, then it is appropriate to prescribe an antibiotic. But other considerations may override the principles of evidence-based medicine: the mother may not be able to come back for a re-examination or the family is about to catch a plane for a holiday etc. Thus, a more holistic approach is mandated and the principle of evidence-based medicine breaks down. There is always a certain unpredictability in our encounters with patients.

Let us take another example. There are many excellent pediatric hospitals that care for patients with cystic fibrosis. A recent article in *The New Yorker* describes how all of them follow the same evidence-based guidelines for the treatment of cystic fibrosis and yet if one examines their results, they are distributed along a bell curve; most of the hospitals were only average in their results and one hospital stood out: the Babies and Children's Hospital in Cleveland where a respirologist named LeRoy Matthews had established a program for the treatment of cystic fibrosis in 1957. When national mortality rates for cystic fibrosis in the best centers was around 20%, Matthews claimed that his mortality rate was less than 2%. What was the difference? The difference turned out to be innovation and constantly challenging the evidence-based guidelines which record past experience.[25] We must remain focused on our patients and challenge ourselves to do better, to go beyond the evidence-based guidelines in order to excel, thereby constantly improving the guidelines themselves.

A recent essay in the New England Journal of Medicine entitled, *The New Language of Medicine* argues that we are in danger of losing the notion that physicians are healers. We now refer to ourselves as 'providers' who have a 'product' to sell and our patients are now 'consumers' buying this product. "Beyond introducing new words, the movement toward industrializing and standardizing all of medicine (rather than just safety and emergency protocols) has caused certain terms that were critical to our medical education to all but disappear. 'Clinical judgment', for instance, is a phrase that has fallen into disgrace, replaced by 'evidence-based practice', the practice of medicine based on scientific data. But evidence is not new; throughout our medical education beginning more than three decades ago, we regularly examined the scientific evidence for our clinical practices. On rounds or in clinical conferences, doctors debated the design and results of numerous research studies. But the exercise of clinical judgment, which permitted assessment of those data and the application of study results to an individual patient, was seen as the acme of professional practice."[26]

In conclusion, there have always been two streams in medicine: the Hippocratic and Aesculapian. Evidence-based medicine and guidelines belong to the Hippocratic stream. The Aesculapian stream emphasizes healing and the importance of the psychological and spiritual aspects involved in healing. Because physicians do not always take this into account, many patients turn to complementary medicine for relief of their symptoms. Modern 21st Century medicine needs to be reminded of both the Hippocratic and the Aesculapian heritage in its long and renowned history. A good physician must take a holistic approach in any clinical encounter with a suffering human being. *Evidence-based medicine must never be abandoned* but it must be incorporated into the practical intellect along with the particular concrete aspects of *this patient* in order to make an appropriate and efficacious therapeutic decision. The cornerstones of caring for our patients and practicing good medicine are the encounter with the patient through our history and physical examination. We then combine this with the principles of evidence-based medicine, recognizing its hermeneutic weakness, to arrive at the best possible outcome for our patient. It is then that evidence-based medicine becomes "'ebullience-based medicine,' a lively, enthusiastic, continually joyful expression of our good fortune at having the privilege to be able to care for and advocate for children."[27]

2. References

[1] Clinicians for the Restoration of Autonomous Practice(CRAP) Writing Group. EBM: unmasking the ugly truth. *BMJ vol. 325, 21-28 December 2002, p1496.*

[2] "A critique of EBM-for example-can be interpreted as being against the best interests of patients and thus against traditional medical ethics. As EBM has become a politically influential doctrine, however, a rational discussion of all sides of EBM is long overdue for the medical profession. Attempts to cover real dilemmas with sarcasm might not facilitate a balanced and useful debate." Saarni,SI,Gylling,HA. Evidence based medicine guidelines: a solution to rationing or politics disguised as science? *J. Med Ethics 2004; 30;p171*

[3] Guyatt G and Rennie D. *Users' guides to the medical literature: essentials of evidence-based practice, p15, November 2002*

[4] Straus,SE, McAlister,FA, Evidence-based medicine: a commentary on common criticisms. *CMAJ,Oct 3,2000;163(7).*

[5] Strauss,SE, McAlister,FA. Evidence-based medicine: a commentary on common criticisms. *CMAJ October 3, 2000; 163(7)p837-841.*

[6] Idem.

[7] Kitchell, J. R., Glover, R.P., and Kyle, R.H. Bilateral internal mammary artery ligation for angina pectoris. *Am J. Cardiol. 1: 46-50, 1958.*

[8] Powell, D. (2011), Atom & cosmos: Hints of a flaw in special relativity: Neutrinos exceed speed of light, but physicists stay skeptical. Science News, 180: 18. doi: 10.1002/scin.5591800920

[9] Frankovich, J et al. Evidence-based medicine in the EMR era. *NEJM, Nov2 2011,p1-2, DOI:10.1056/NEJMp1108726*

[10] Ibid.p2

[11] Vineis,P. Evidence-based medicine and ethics: a practical approach. *J. Med Ethics 2004; 30;126-130;p126130.*

[12] Slowther,A, Ford, S,Schofield,T. Ethics of evidence based medicine in the primary care setting. *J. Med Ethics 2004;30;151-155.*

[13] Nissen SE, Wolski,K. Effect of rosiglitazone on the risk of myocardial infarction and death from cardiovascular causes. *NEJM 2007; 356: 2457-71.*

[14] Ioannidis JPA. Why most published research findings are false. *PloS Medicine. Volume 2, Issue 8,e024, 696-701, August 2005.*

[15] Olivieri NF, Brittenham GM, McLaren CE, et al. Long term safety and effectiveness of iron chelation therapy with deferiprone for thalassemia major. *NEJM 1998; 339;417-23.*

[16] Viens AM, Savulescu J. Introduction to the Olivieri symposium. *J Med Ethics 2004;30;1-7*

[17] Bomardier C et al. Comparison of upper gastrointestinal toxicity of rofecoxib and naproxren in patients with rheumatoid arthritis. *NEJM 343, No 21,November 23, 2000, p152-15280.*

Mukherjee D, Nissen SE, Topol EJ. Risk of cardiovascular events associated with selective COX-2 inhibitors . *JAMA, August 22/29,2001,Vol 286, No8, p954-959*

[18] De Angelis C et al, Clinical trial registration: a statement from the International Committee of Medical Journal Editors. *The Lancet. Vol. 364. issue 9438, p911-912, 2004.*

Clinical trial registration: a statement from the International Committee of Medical Journal Editors. Editorial. C. De Angelis et al. *New England Journal of Medicine, Volume 351Number 12, p1250-1251, September 16, 2004.*

[19] Gamble VN. Under the shadow of Tuskegee: African Americans and health care. *Amer J of Public Health November 1997, vol.87, no.11. p17731778.*

[20] Shevell M. Hallervorden and history. *NEJM 348;1; January 2, 2003, p3-4.*

[21] Wakefield ,AJ et al. Ileal-lymphoid-nodular hyperplasia, non-specific colitis, and pervasive developmental disorder in children. *Lancet 351:37,641, 1998.*

[22] Deer, B. How the case against the MMR vaccine was fixed. *BMJ, vol 342, January 8, 2011, p77.*

[23] Editors of the Lancet. Retraction: ileal lymphoid nodular hyperplasia, non-specific colitis, and pervasive developmental disorder in children. *Lancet* 2010;375:445.

[24] Increased transmission and outbreaks of measles-European region, 2011. *Morbidity and Mortality Weekly Report(MMWR), Dec. 2, 2011/60(47);1605-1610.*

[25] Gawande A. The bell curve. *The New Yorker,December 6, 2004.*
[26] Hartzband P and Groopman J. The new language of medicine. *NEJM, 365;15,October13 2011, p1372*
[27] Callahan,CW. Observations of an older pediatrician: supplementing evidence-based medicine. *Pediatrics in Review, Vol 22, No 9, 293-294, September 2001. .*

10

EBM in Clinical Practice: Implementation in Osteopathic Diagnosis and Manipulative Treatment for Non-Specific Low Back Pain Patients

Rafael Zegarra-Parodi, Jerry Draper-Rodi,
Laurent Fabre, Julien Bardin and Pauline Allamand
Osteopaths, Private Practice,
France

1. Introduction

1.1 Non-specific low back pain in western countries

Low back pain (LBP) is an extremely common problem which most people in industrialized countries experience at some point in their lives. The prevalence of LBP in the USA ranges from 8% to 56% (Manchikanti, 2000). Estimation of the one-year incidence of a first-ever episode of LBP ranges between 6.3% and 15.4%, while estimation of the one-year incidence of any episode of LBP ranges between 1.5% and 36%. Studies have found the incidence of LBP is highest in the third decade, and overall prevalence increases with age up to the 60-65 year age group, and then gradually declines. Many environmental and personal factors influence the onset and course of LBP. In addition to age, commonly reported risk factors include low educational status, stress, anxiety, depression, professional dissatisfaction, low levels of social support in the workplace and whole-body vibration activities. LBP has an enormous impact on individuals, families, communities, governments and businesses throughout the world (Hoy et al, 2010), and associated costs are estimated at between between $20 billion and $50 billion per year (Nachemson, 1992).

Non-specific low back pain (NS-LBP) represents about 85% of LBP patients seen in primary care (Deyo and Phillips, 1996), and the vast majority of LBP patients seen by physical therapists are classified under this label. This classification process differentiates between specific spinal pathology, nerve root pain and simple or NS-LBP (Waddell, 2004). Patients suffering from NS-LBP who are not improving may benefit from referral for spinal manipulation provided by a trained spinal care specialist such as a physical therapist, chiropractor, osteopathic physician or physician who specializes in musculoskeletal medicine (NGC-7704, 2009). No evidence was found to support recommending regular manipulative treatment for the prevention of LBP (NGC-7704, 2009). High-quality evidence suggests that there is no clinically relevant difference between the efficacy of spinal manipulative therapy (SMT) and other interventions for reducing pain and improving function in patients with chronic NS-LBP. Determining cost-effectiveness of care is of high priority (Rubinstein et al,

2011). Risk of serious complications after spinal manipulation is low (estimated risk: cauda equina syndrome, less than one in one million). Current guidelines contraindicate manipulation on people with severe or progressive neurological deficit (NGC-7704, 2009).

1.2 Osteopathy and osteopathic medicine

In the USA, osteopathic physicians are licensed to practise the full scope of medicine. In Europe, Australia and New-Zealand, osteopaths are first-contact practitioners trained in private or academic institutions with Bachelors or Masters degree levels, and they are allowed to provide only osteopathic manipulative treatment (OMT) (WHO Benchmarks, 2010). OMT is one of the numerous treatment approaches within manual and manipulative therapies for the management of a variety of musculoskeletal and non-musculoskeletal conditions. A wide range of manual techniques described in the *Authorized Osteopathic Thesaurus (AOT)* (Authorized Osteopathic Thesaurus, 2009) are used for the treatment of somatic dysfunction (SD). A SD is a functional disturbance of the musculoskeletal system tissues and related vascular and neurological components (Rumney, 1975). Osteopathic care relies on four tenets: (1) the body is a unit; the person is a unit of body, mind, and spirit, (2) the body is capable of self-regulation, self-healing, and health maintenance, (3) structure and function are reciprocally interrelated and (4) rational treatment is based upon an understanding of the basic principles of body unity, self-regulation, and the interrelationship of structure and function (Rogers et al, 2002).

The distinguishing features of osteopathic care described in the scientific literature seem to be the concept of SD, the OMT and the four basic tenets of osteopathic therapeutic principles (WHO Benchmarks, 2010). Although these concepts were proposed mainly for educational purposes, they appear to be central in osteopathic practice, and are currently challenged by evidence-informed osteopathy (Fryer, 2008).

The SD is a pathological entity referenced in the International Classifications of Diseases (ICD) 10 and has a political use as a tool distinctive from other manual therapies (Zegarra-Parodi, 2010). This concept relies however on biomechanical and neurophysiological theories that are partially supported in clinical practice. It is recommended to osteopathic physicians to use OMT for NS-LBP caused by musculoskeletal conditions, i.e. to treat SD related to LBP (NGC-7504, 2009).

OMT is a distinctive therapeutic modality which significantly decreases LBP with an effect size of -0.30 (CI 95% = [-0.47;-0.13]). The level of pain reduction is greater than expected from placebo effects alone and persists for at least three months (Licciardone et al, 2005a).

1.3 Purpose

The purpose of this chapter is to describe current clinical and scientific evidence regarding the concept of somatic dysfunction associated with non-specific low back pain for osteopathic manipulative diagnosis and treatment. This clinical concept will be analyzed in the light of evidence-based medicine.

2. Methods

A systematic literature search was conducted in July 2011 to identify published papers examining osteopathic manipulative diagnosis and treatment of NS-LBP patients. The research included studies from 1975 onwards, i.e. since SD was first defined by Rumney. The databases searched were Medline, CINAHL and the Cochrane library. The search terms were as follows: key term - "somatic dysfunction", "low back pain", "osteopathic manipulative treatment" or "OMT" "osteopathic diagnosis". The key terms were searched for in the title, abstract and keywords. Studies were included if they were written in English or French. The reference lists of retrieved studies were scanned to identify additional relevant papers.

3. Results

3.1 Osteopathic diagnosis: The somatic dysfunction concept

3.1.1 Historical aspects

Littlejohn, one of the pioneers of osteopathy, developed the concept of physiological disturbance associated with mechanical strain from the bony structures in 1903. He suggested that a properly functioning nervous system was a key element to maintain health and recover from disease. Burns then began to study physiological effects following manipulations at the Kirksville College of Osteopathic Medicine (KCOM) in the early 20th century. She mapped the effects produced by osteopathic lesions - manipulable lesions described by osteopaths - at different spinal segments, and found a close correspondence in the pattern produced in experiments on animals and the clinical patterns observed in herself and her colleagues (Allan, 1986). Experimental studies suggested the involvement of the parasympathetic and the sympathetic pathways in the genesis of the osteopathic lesion through viscerosomatic reflexes (Burns, 1948). Denslow and Korr (Denslow, 1993; Korr, 1997) from KCOM led the first experimental studies on the human body to lend support to a model providing a neurological explanation for the origin and maintenance of the osteopathic lesion. They observed paraspinal muscle hyperexcitability associated with two misaligned vertebrae and alteration of sympathetic nervous system activity through sudomotricity studies. Some musculoskeletal symptoms quickly improved with manipulation: the nervous system is the only system that can operate almost instantaneously and may therefore be the mechanism behind the effects seen following manipulation. They developed the "facilitated segment" concept (Korr, 1979): an injured somatic or visceral structure produces discordant afferent impulses creating what is now described as a sensitization of the dorsal horn. The osteopathic lesion was initially described according to its characteristic features: altered range and quality of joint movement, altered tissue texture in the surrounding tissues, and sometimes apparent asymmetry of one vertebra compared to the others (Korr, 1947).

Rumney, from the KCOM, wrote the first paper describing the concept of SD (Rumney, 1975). Three major components of disease had been identified: visceral, psychic and somatic. He focused on the somatic component. He thought that the osteopathic profession had misled other health professions about what osteopathy was, by introducing the adjective "osteopathic" to terms, as in "osteopathic lesion" or "osteopathic pathology", creating difficulties communicating with other scientific groups. Inaccurate concepts used by early osteopaths for manipulations such as the "bone out of place" were then replaced by concepts focusing more on the physiopathological consequences of biomechanical impairments as scientific knowledge increased within the osteopathic profession. The SD was therefore defined as *"an area of impaired function of related components of the musculoskeletal system (muscle, bone, fascia and ligament) and its associated or related parts in the vascular, lymphatic, and nervous systems"*. Three important criteria for manual diagnosis were described: tissue changes, hyperalgesia and motion changes. This diagnosis is based on different signs in order to lead to a precise treatment, making specific adjustments. This concept was a shift from previous theories, which held that a global approach was sufficient to be effective.

In 1990 Van Buskirk, an American osteopath, came up with a model to support the SD pathogenesis (Van Buskirk, 1990). This model focused on nociceptors, as they were the only described sensory receptors which could generate muscle hypertonia, autonomic arousal, and consequent loco-regional circulatory impairments commonly associated with SD. Van Buskirk's SD model brought together three previous models based on: changes in nervous system activity, in connective tissue and in local circulation. Nervous system activity changes associated with SD corresponded to an increase of sympathetic outflow caused by localized excessive nociceptive information from visceral or somatic structures. Maintaining excessive nociceptive input would be detrimental to the normal function of the organ involved, and immune function would theoretically be diminished. These afferents would also produce reflex muscle contraction by axon reflex and sympathetic vasodilatation effects which would engorge the affected muscles and produce a restriction of motion. Over time, the muscle would become fibrotic and if stretched or strained again, nociceptors would be activated once again.

3.1.2 Physiological studies

Fryer, from Victoria University, Australia, recently revisited the SD neurophysiological theories with modern equipment (Fryer, 1999; Fryer, 2003), focusing on paraspinal tissue texture changes detected with palpation associated with electromyographic (EMG) data. A literature review has shown that the concept of reactive muscle contraction associated with intervertebral dysfunction seems plausible (Fryer et al, 2004a). The deep paraspinal muscle inhibition observed during dynamic and static activities was used as a theoretical framework for a possible relationship between dysfunctional muscle activity and tissue texture change findings with SD. However abnormal paraspinal tissues detected with palpation were associated with increased and/or decreased muscle activity (Fryer et al, 2004b). They then tried to find a possible relationship between an abnormal paraspinal muscle palpation and local sensitivity measured using an algometer. They observed that paraspinal sites identified as having abnormal tissue texture and tenderness diagnosed by palpation, had significantly lower mean pressure pain threshold than other sites immediately surrounding the abnormal region (Fryer et al, 2004c). These results tend to corroborate common palpation findings diagnosed by osteopathic practitioners. Increased motor activity might be a contributing factor to tissue changes detected with palpation (Fryer et al, 2006).

Fryer pursued his studies at the Andrew Taylor Still Research Institute (ATSRI) in Kirksville where Korr and Denslow had worked 60 years before. Principal biases, i.e. thinner intramuscular wires, proper statistical analysis and limited cohort size, were corrected. Recent studies concluded that there was no evidence of distinguishing EMG activity in the deep thoracic paraspinal musculature at sites identified as abnormal to palpation under resting conditions, compared to sites identified as normal (Fryer et al, 2010a). They suggested that other factors than muscle activity, such as tissue fluid and inflammatory mediators, could be responsible for the apparent abnormality of these tissues during palpation.

3.2 Osteopathic palpatory findings in LBP patients

The SD concept underlies the diagnosis and the treatment in osteopathic medicine in clinical guidelines. In the USA, the National Guideline Clearinghouse (NGC) recommended that OMT be utilized by osteopathic physicians to treat SD associated with NS-LBP (NGC-7504, 2009). This recommendation has a 1a level of evidence (the highest level) and is based on the results of a systematic review of randomized controlled trials (Licciardone et al, 2005a).

Fundamental requirements for a diagnostic test to be recommended to clinicians are its accuracy and its reliability (Bossuyt et al, 2003). Over recent years, evidence-based medicine has challenged osteopathic practicioners to favor proven reliable palpatory tests when diagnosing patients' conditions. Determining the accuracy and reliability of diagnostic tests used in osteopathy is therefore a high priority (Lucas and Bogduk, 2010). For that purpose, the ATSRI tried to investigate the interobserver reliability of common osteopathic palpatory tests used to evaluate the lumbar spine (Degenhardt et al, 2005). Three practitioners performed common palpatory tests for the clinical findings associated with SD: tenderness, tissue texture changes, vertebral positional asymmetry, and motion asymmetry in subjects. The procedure was repeated and the results were re-evaluated after consensus training had been completed by the examiners. This study showed that the initial evaluation of interobserver reliability for the four tests was poor to fair (kappa ranged from -0.02 to 0.34). Acceptable kappa values for clinical tests were achieved after consensus training only for tissue texture and tenderness, but the tenderness test was the only test that had a good kappa value (k=0.68).

The lack of reliable tests in manual medicine is common as there is no gold standard except for pain. Acceptable reliability in diagnosing SD could however be achieved with appropriate and regular training in clinical studies and then be recommended to clinicians. Snider et al. (2008) investigated the incidence and severity of SD of four lumbar vertebral segments (L1-L4) in subjects with chronic NS-LBP. They included 16 subjects with chronic LBP and 47 subjects without chronic LBP. Subjects' four lumbar vertebral segments (L1-L4) were evaluated. From 15 palpatory tests taught at KCOM, the four that achieved greatest inter-examiner reliability in the Degenhardt et al. study (2005) were included in a specific training protocol designed to promote consensus between examiners. The two groups showed significantly different severity of SD, determined from tissue texture changes ($p=0.006$) and static rotational asymmetry ($p=0.008$). Severity was found to be greater for the chronic LBP group than for the non-LBP group. Significant differences were observed in the incidence of vertebrae testing positive for resistance to anterior springing ($p<0.001$) and tenderness ($p=0.002$), with both occurring more frequently in the chronic LBP group than in the non-LBP group. Furthermore, the severity of SD as determined with resistance to anterior springing ($p<0.001$) and tenderness ($p=0.001$) was also significantly different between the two groups, with the chronic LBP group again showing greater severity than the non-LBP group. NS-LBP patients have more severe SD compared to asymptomatic patients and clinicians usually associate these clinical findings with symptoms to shape specific OMT for each patient. Snider et al. (2010) investigated the association of lumbar SD as assessed with palpation with bone mineral density (BMD) among LBP and healthy patients. They observed that lumbar segments with palpated rotational asymmetry had higher mean BMD T scores than lumbar segments with no asymmetry ($p=0.002$). Lumbar segments with anterior motion restriction had higher mean BMD T scores than lumbar segments with no motion restriction ($p=0.03$). LBP patients demonstrated higher regional mean lumbar BMD T scores than those without LBP ($p<0.001$). These results suggest an association of objective lumbar vertebral BMD variation to palpatory findings associated with SD.

Although patients describe the same symptoms, OMT is test-dependent and then specific according to SD incidence and severity, and the association made with symptoms by the practitioner. Pain provocation tests are currently described as the most reliable, and soft tissue paraspinal palpatory diagnostic tests and landmarks as not reliable. Practitioners should therefore combine their own experience with current data to select specific tests in order to achieve a precise SD diagnosis.

3.3 Osteopathic Manipulative Treatment for LBP patients

It has now been established that SD can be treated by OMT (Fryer, 1999) and several studies describe the benefits of OMT in the treatment of LBP (Licciardone et al, 2005a). However even if scientific evidence supporting the effectiveness of OMT has emerged, there is still a lack of scientific evidence to describe the psycho-physiological mechanisms underlying these treatments (Evans, 2002).

The main explanations for the effects of manual techniques are based on data from human and animal studies, and recent models rely on neurophysiology (Pickar, 2002; Skyba et al, 2003). Manipulation-induced hypoalgesia has been demonstrated in studies with human subjects (Sterling et al, 2001). Skyba et al. (2003) demonstrated in an experimental study on rats, that the antihyperalgesia produced by joint manipulation appears to involve descending inhibitory mechanisms which utilize serotonin and norepinephrine. Pickar (2002) explained that spinal manipulation impacts proprioceptive primary afferent neurons from paraspinal tissues, paraspinal tissues. He suggested that this can affect pain processing, possibly by altering the central facilitated state of the spinal cord, the motor control system, and through somato-somatic reflex and somato-visceral reflex. Several studies have shown a relationship between spinal manipulation and response of the autonomic nervous system (ANS): spinal manipulation induced a sympathetic response that was measured by the modification of skin conductance or the α-amylase-activity (Sterling et al, 2001; Henderson et al, 2010) and OMT produced vagal response (Henley et al, 2008).

Several studies (Sherman et al, 2004; Andersson et al, 1999; Licciardone et al, 2003) describe OMT's beneficial effects on symptoms of chronic pain patients. For NS-LBP patients in particular, Degenhardt et al (2007) observed a decrease in pain blood markers associated with a decreased level of stress described by patients 24 hours after receiving OMT.

3.4 Osteopathic diagnosis and Osteopathic Manipulative Treatment records in a clinical setting

Despite the SD's ICD classification (ICD-10, 2007), the SD nomenclature is not universally used: a 2010 study of the UK osteopathic profession revealed multiple terms used to describe this palpatory diagnosis of "somatic dysfunction", including "restriction", "naming by anatomical aetiology", "dysfunction", "facet lock", "motion restriction" and more than 12 other names (Fryer, 2010b). Despite the lack of uniform terminology for the SD, the Louisa Burns Osteopathic Research Committee of the American Academy of Osteopathy standardized the palpatory diagnosis of SD by developing and validating the Outpatient Osteopathic Subjective Objective Assessment Plan Note Form Series (OOSNF). These data records sheets are standardized and used to objectively measure and record the diagnosis and treatment of SD during patient encounters (Sleszynski et al, 1999). Two systematic reviews (Seffinger et al, 2004; Stochkendahl et al, 2006) recommended that clinicians should not base their diagnosis on a single clinical examination such as palpation, but rather on a range of tests and findings (Brunse al, 2010). The SD diagnosis is not used in a pain and movement model as in manual medicine for example, but includes other previously described clinical findings. Its four diagnostic criteria are commonly represented in the osteopathic literature by the acronym TART: **(T)** tissue texture abnormality: effusions, laxity, stability, tone; **(A)** asymmetry: crepitation, defects, masses, misalignment; **(R)** restriction of motion: contracture and **(T)** tenderness: pain (Outpatient Osteopathic SOAP Note Form, 2002; Authorized Osteopathic Thesaurus, 2009).

The OOSNF musculoskeletal table is used to collect data on the musculoskeletal evaluation of 13 anatomic regions: head, cervical, upper thoracic (T1–T4), midthoracic (T5–T9), lower thoracic (T10–T12), lumbar, sacrum/pelvis, pelvis/innominate, lower extremities (left and right), upper extremities (left and right), and ribs. For each of the patient's anatomic regions, the osteopathic practitioner evaluates the severity of SD. The scoring criteria for levels of SD are as follows: (0 - None): no SD present or background levels of SD only, (1 - Mild): more than background levels of SD, minor TART elements present, (2 - Moderate): obvious TART elements, which may or may not be overtly symptomatic, with significant restriction of motion and/or tenderness elements present and (3 - Severe): key SD with significant symptomatology, including restriction of motion and/or tenderness elements that "stand out" with minimal search or provocation (Sleszynski et al, 1999).

Johnson and Kurtz (2003) classified OMT in three categories: (1) direct techniques which engage the restrictive barrier: articulatory, High-Velocity Low-Amplitude Thrust (HVLAT), muscle energy, soft tissue, (2) indirect techniques applied away from the restrictive barrier: counterstain, cranial, facilitated positional release, functional, fascial ligamentous release, and (3) direct-indirect techniques: myofascial/integrated neuromuscular release, lymphatic. The OMT modalities used to treat the SD evaluated in correlation with the patient chief complaint and the perception of how the SD in each region responded to OMT immediately after treatment are reported. The scoring criteria for responses after OMT are either: (R) Resolved: the SD is completely resolved without evidence of it ever having been present, (I) Improved: the SD is improved but not completely resolved, (U) Unchanged: the SD is unchanged or the same after treatment as it was before treatment, (W) Worse: the SD is worse or aggravated immediately after treatment. In the final section, the osteopathic practitioner details new medications, exercises he wishes the patient to carry out and nutritional, food or diet recommendations (Outpatient Osteopathic SOAP Note Form, 2002).

Members of the profession should consider the long-term value of this widely accessible database which will facilitate descriptive and clinical osteopathic studies (Sleszynski and Glonek, 2005). These tools, which have been used in published research are necessary for the osteopathic profession's future, as governments and paying third-parties require more evidence to justify treatment reimbursement. The profession has the opportunity to provide data to describe, explain, and support OMT's effectiveness for musculoskeletal and non-musculoskeletal conditions.

3.5 Osteopathic management of LBP patients: Patient-practitioner interaction

The emphasis in treating patients who have NS-LBP is on improving function, decreasing peripheral nociception and central facilitation, and empowering individuals to move forward in resuming their normal daily life activities (Kuchera, 2005).

A growing number of chronic pain patients are consulting complementary and alternative medicine (CAM) practitioners owing to dissatisfaction with mainstream medicine. (Kuchera, 2007) Patients appreciate having an individual answer to their symptoms, and an understandable explanation. As diagnosis in osteopathic medicine is not based only on pain, patients presenting the same symptoms may not receive the same treatment. Each osteopathic practitioner designs a specific treatment according to the patient's expectations and his/her osteopathic diagnosis, i.e. the SDs relating to the NS-LBP. The test-dependant OMT for SD may focus on various local, spinal and supra-spinal theoretical outcomes determining technique choices and goals. OMT is chosen and adapted after obtaining patients' consent, and treatment strategies depend on the patient's ability to face the treatment's homeostatic response and the main underlying pathophysiological mechanism (Kuchera, 2007).

Lifestyle and habits, including ergonomics, are crucial points to take into consideration as they may be provoking or sustaining factors for SD, and can challenge treatment results or even prevent amelioration. Patient history should therefore encompass these aspects and look carefully for possible personal or occupational biomechanical stressors. Such information could be included in a specific patient education programme in order to avoid dysfunctional strain patterns leading to recurrent symptoms.

According to Kuchera (2007), physical examination of chronic pain patients by osteopathic practitioners should not be limited to searching for pain generators, as chronic pain is often associated with anxiety, depression and a reduction in the quality of life. Chronic pain shifts pain activity from the sensory cortex to the anterior cingulate gyrus, leading patients to describe their suffering rather than the location of their pain. Osteopathic practitioners use patient communication about social, family and emotional impact of illness rather than focusing on pain (Carey et al, 2003) and provide health and diet advice (Kuchera, 2007).

An American study showed that the length of consultation was longer for osteopathic physicians compared to allopathic physicians: 20 minutes versus 15 minutes on average ($p<0.01$) (Sun et al, 2004). This feature may have a positive therapeutic influence on the perception and understanding of pain by the patient, which is described as a possible psychosocial risk factor for transition from acute to chronic pain (Penney, 2010). Quality of care and patient satisfaction with osteopathic practitioners could be attributed to communication and empathy (Pincus et al, 2000).

4. Discussion

4.1 Osteopathic diagnosis for LBP patients

The International Association for the Study of Pain (IASP) describes two main models to explain LBP's physiopathological mechanisms: the End-Organ Dysfunction Model (EODM) and the Altered Nervous System Processing Models (ANSPM) (Pain, Clinical Updates: Low Back Pain, 2010). Both models are for educational and treatment purposes; it is supposed that treatment is more effective if it targets specific physiopathological mechanisms. The EODM supports the theory that nociceptive stimuli are caused by lumbar spine pathologies such as injuries, degenerative changes or repetitive strain injuries. However LBP does not always correlate with lumbar spine pathologies diagnosed by MRI scans or pain provocation/palliation techniques. It is proposed in the ANSPM that perception of sensory information is altered. This alteration might be due to physiological changes within the nervous system with an increased susceptibility to pain due to psychological vulnerabilities, such as depression or anxiety. In daily practice, practitioners reported that patients suffering from LBP are predisposed to reporting additional chronic pain syndromes. Researchers have discovered that sensory neurons, usually silent in healthy patients, may become reorganized and generate spontaneous action potentials leading to a rewiring of the central nervous system in chronic pain conditions. However symptoms described by LBP patients cannot be explained with a single model but rather with a combination of EODM and ANSPM with variation for each patient. It is interesting to observe that the clinical concept of SD combines these two approaches, i.e. a biomechanical strain from somatic and visceral structures which is associated with altered reflexive neurological responses from the involved anatomical area to the spinal cord.

SD diagnosed among NS-LBP patients may be causative, reflexive, reactive or perpetuating, or a mix of these. Models for SD are controversial and rely on biomechanics (Triano, 2001) and neurophysiological reflexes (Van Buskirk, 1990; Pickar, 2002; Howell and Willard, 2005). Data from scientific literature about mechanical and neurophysiological modifications observed in LBP patients may also be interpreted by osteopathic practitioners using the SD concept, but this does not give a scientific validation of this concept. Here are two examples of results from EMG and ulstrasonography studies on LBP patients where the results could be "osteopathically" interpreted, i.e. focusing not only on local physiopathological changes but also looking at possible interactions with other anatomical areas according to their biomechanical and neurophysiological functions. Some of these physiopathological changes could also be associated with palpatory findings by experienced practitioners and be interpreted using the concept of SD to improve osteopathic diagnosis.

In a comparative study, Van Dieën et al. (2003) revisited conflicting evidence on the modified activity of trunk muscles in NS-LBP patients. The main theory was based on a pain-spasm-pain model where it was considered that pain was generating muscle activity which in turn caused pain. This model was supported by EMG activity found during motor tasks: increased activity of antagonist muscles, decreased activity of agonist muscles, and no increased activity in static posture. However Van Dieën et al. highlighted that previous studies demonstrated disparate results caused by methodological flaws especially in the normalization of EMG data. After improving the standardization of the EMG baseline, they measured the activities of agonist and antagonist trunk muscles during trunk motions in healthy and LBP patients. EMG ratios between lumbar and thoracic erector spinae were calculated and they observed that trunk muscle use in patients with LBP was greater than in healthy control subjects. They suggested a trunk muscle strategy aiming to increase spinal stability in LBP patients.

It has been hypothesized that the connective tissues forming the fascial planes of the back play a role in the pathogenesis of chronic LBP. In a randomized trial, Langevin et al. (2009) observed that LBP patients had, on average, 25% greater perimuscular connective tissue thickness than did subjects without LBP. According to these authors, increased thickness and disorganization of connective tissue layers due to inflammation, fatty infiltration, fibrosis and adhesions may impair the normal relative movement of connective tissue planes, increase tissue stiffness, decrease range of motion and predispose to further injury. Disorganized connective tissue layers may also cause pain due to trapping of sensory nerve fibres through the collagen matrix.

4.2 Osteopathic Manipulative Treatment for LBP patients: Implications for treatment

Licciardone, Brimhall and King from the Osteopathic Research Center (ORC) carried out a systematic review and meta-analysis of randomised clinical trials on OMT for LBP (Licciardone et al 2005a). The effects of SMT on LBP patients were already reported in the literature but no data was available to evaluate the specific OMT on that patient population. Spinal manipulations and mobilizations are effective in adults for acute, subacute LBP and for chronic LBP (Bronfort et al, 2010).

Eight OMT studies versus control treatments were included in their meta-analysis. They were conducted between 1973 and 2001 in the USA and the UK. They met good methodology quality criteria. The methodological quality of four of the OMT trials was independently confirmed in a recent systematic review which included a best evidence synthesis incorporating eight explicit quality criteria, including similarity of baseline characteristics of subjects or reporting of adjusted outcomes; concealment of treatment allocation; blinding of subjects; blinding of providers or other control for attention bias; blinded or unbiased outcomes assessment; subject dropouts being reported and accounted for in the analysis; missing data being reported and accounted for in the analysis; and intention-to-treat analysis or absence of differential co-interventions between groups in studies with full compliance.

Two out of the three authors reviewed the articles independently, and conflicting data were resolved by consensus. Effect size computed with Cohen's d statistic was used to report all trial results. Effect size is the measure of the strength of the relationship between two variables in a statistical population. The negative effect found size represented a greater decrease in pain among OMT subjects relative to control treatment subjects.

This meta-analysis included 525 subjects with LBP from the 8 eligible trials. Pain associated with OMT was very significantly reduced. Analysis was performed with a best-case and a worse-case scenario. Both supported the efficacy of OMT for LBP, and showed an improved reduction in pain with OMT in comparison with placebo control or active treatment, though the worst-case scenario was not found to be statistically significant. LBP symptoms treated with OMT were significantly reduced in the short-term (effect size, -0.28; 95% CI, -0.51 to -0.06; $p = 0.01$), medium-term (effect size, -0.33; 95% CI, -0.51 to -0.15; $p < 0.001$), and long-term (effect size, -0.40; 95% CI, -0.74 to -0.05; $p = 0.03$) follow-up periods. Overall results showed a statistically significant reduction in LBP in patients treated with OMT. Stratified meta-analyses were performed to control for moderator variables, and this showed that OMT significantly reduced low back pain versus active treatment / placebo control and versus no treatment control. OMT might act as a substitute for, or decrease the use of, medication known to carry risks of substantial side-effects. Contrary to the USA, osteopaths in the UK are not licensed physicians. Effect sizes observed in the UK study were comparable to those found in the USA studies suggesting that the results reflected accurately the effects of OMT and not other elements of low back care.

Systematic imaging prior to OMT is not part of professional guidelines, but its absence may limit the differential diagnosis process, and prohibit the use of some potentially iatrogenic OMT. The most serious adverse effects of manual techniques are vertebral artery dissections following cervical manipulations (Vogel, 2010). A systematic review of the literature on the side effects of manual therapies (Carnes et al, 2010) concluded that severe side effects were low but half of patients described post-manipulative transient mild to moderate side effects. Patients treated by final year students in a clinical center integrated in a UK osteopathic school were surveyed about the main side-effects experienced after OMT (Rajendran et al, 2009). Patients consulted primarily for LBP (33%) and neck pain (20%). Local pain (24.3%), local stiffness (18,3%), and an increase in the pain that motivated the consultation (11.8%) were the most common side-effects reported. They were felt up to two days after the consultation but 96% of these manifestations were considered by the patients as mild or moderate.

The numbers of OMT sessions for LBP patients reported varies in the literature (Licciardone et al, 2005a): treatment protocols included from 4 to 10 sessions lasting from 15 to 45 minutes over a period of one to six months. The authors did not reference or justify their choices for the protocol which were mainly based on experts' opinions. However, the format most consistent with current clinical practice would be around 6 to 8 sessions with a frequency of one session every 2 weeks over a period of 3 to 4 months.

Sloan and Walsh (2010) demonstrated how the language used by practitioners could affect patients' pain perception and outcomes among LBP patients. Mechanical explanations about patients' conditions were associated with better outcomes than degenerative ones. Placebo responses are often described pejoratively and interpreted as something administered to patients which cannot be controlled, but the patient's response is nonetheless a positive one. Nocebo responses may result from words used by practitioners while talking with their patients to describe their conditions. Practitioners should keep in mind the possible iatrogenic effects of their vocabulary, and should use simple and neutral words in order to give patients an explanation that makes sense to them. As with all other healthcare practitioners, the placebo response could therefore be enhanced, and depends mainly on how osteopathic practitioners describe their understanding of the symptoms. This affects patients' beliefs about prognosis and attitudes towards treatment and self-care (Abbey, 2011).

4.3 Osteopathic Manipulative Treatment for LBP patients: Implications for training

Palpation teaching presents specific challenges. Four main issues have been described in the scientific literature surrounding manual therapies, and should be addressed to improve palpation teaching: hand positioning, amount and direction of force and interpretation of tissue response (Degenhardt, 2009). Educators in osteopathy train students to perform techniques and to adapt them according to patient needs in a clinical context, to describe relative and absolute contraindications, and to describe expected outcomes. The typical lecturing process is to teach OMT every year from the first year, gradually teaching more complicated and refined methods to develop students' skills (Standard 2000: Standard of proficiency March 1999. General Osteopathic Council (GOsC), 2000).

Osteopathic training within universities now includes a sound background to the biomechanical and neurophysiological aspects of OMT. Theoretical models of action are currently shifting away from a classical mechanistic view to a systemic view, incorporating data from recent publications. Different models of practice in osteopathy have been described: biomechanical, neurological, respiratory/circulatory, behavioral/psychological and bioenergetic models (WHO Benchmarks, 2010). They differ regarding the application of forces and comprehension of the body's response to mechanical and psychological stresses. Palpatory findings associated with SD may vary according to the theoretical model, and this may create cognitive conflicts (Johsua and Dupin, 1993). Diversity of concepts requiring different cognitive and manual approaches may be a source of confusion for students. Some osteopathic education centres have therefore prioritized SD and OMT theoretical and practical training according to their scientific levels of evidence. Manipulation and mobilization were therefore prioritized probably because they are better supported by current evidence. This is probably because these direct OMTs are similar to techniques performed and studied by other professionals (Lederman, 2005). Direct OMTs use mainly biomechanical (Triano, 2001) and neurophysiological models (Van Buskirk, 1990; Pickar, 2002; Howell and Willard, 2005).

Clinimetrics is the practice of assessing or describing symptoms, signs and laboratory findings by means of scales, indices and other quantitative instruments (Feinstein, 1987). It is clinically important to focus on this during training in order to train future professionals to make appropriate decisions about patient management, based on the best level of evidence available. A clinical measurement instrument, such as a test, should ideally be *valid* (it should measure what it is intended to measure), be *reliable*, i.e. reproducible (the instrument score should remain stable when there has been no change in the performance), be *responsive* to change over time, and be *precise* enough to measure the minimal clinically important change (MIC), defined by Jaeschke et al (2009) as the smallest difference in score in the domain of interest which patients perceive as beneficial, and which would mandate, in the absence of troublesome side effects and excessive cost, a change in the patient's management. These challenging aspects have been assessed for osteopathy osteopathy. As with as with other manual therapies, not having gold standards to evaluate tests with to assess their validity is a problem (Lucas and Bogduk, 2011). Studies assessing diagnostic reliability should be standardized, and under ideal conditions conditions, have certain variables controlled, the most important being that the examiners should be blinded to other examiners' findings for inter-examiner reliability studies. The application and interpretation of the test should be appropriate and there should be enough time between repeated measurements to avoid altering results.

Osteopathic educators should prioritize the contents of their training programmes according to the tests' performances. Tests should also be, as stated above, valid, responsive to change over time, such as before and after treatment, and precise enough to measure the MIC. Insufficient performance of tests in the detection of MIC may cause a type-2 error in RCTs; no difference is observed during the study when in reality there is a difference between groups (Lucas and Bogduk, 2011). Students should also be aware of such limitations of studies during critical appraisal of published literature in the manual therapies field.

4.4 Evidence-oriented osteopathy

EBM has been defined by Sackett et al. (1996) as "the conscientious, explicit, and judicious use of current best evidence in making decisions about the care of individual patients". Incorporation of EBM in daily practice for clinicians is a challenging issue, especially for manual therapists therapists, owing to the lack of reliable and valid tests excepting, the pain reproduction tests. Evidence based medicine cannot however be "cookbook" medicine because each patient is a unique individual with different medical needs (ATSU, Evidence Based Medicine, 2011). For example, the main pathophysiological mechanisms underlying a patient's symptoms or injury might be evaluated through case history: sclerotomal tissue pain described as "deep, dull, or toothache-like", and myotomal pain that is difficult to localise and is described as "crampy" or "stiff" (Kuchera, 2007). Discussing the generalizability of published data also requires critical appraisal skills that are common to all other healthcare professionals, and osteopathic practitioners should ask themselves if results from research are applicable specifically to their patients. Interpretation of such studies has, however, several limitations. The main one is that osteopathy should be considered as a complex intervention (Sturmberg and Martin, 2008), and needs to be evaluated using specific methodological tools which are different for pharmacological interventions.

A scope of practice for osteopathic practitioners is about to be published in Europe (European Federation of Osteopaths (EFO), The Scope of Osteopathic Practice in Europe, 2011). Osteopaths themselves have defined the indication for OMT as the presence of SD that is clinically significant. The SD concept may however be perceived as perverted by part of the profession when used as a tool to categorize their patients, rather than a tool to diagnose and treat them (Johnson and Kurtz, 2003). This concept has caused the profession to lose part of its monistic vision (Lee, 2005), by implying a direct link between SD and symptoms and diseases, which in reality corresponds to a biomedical model (Leigh, 1994)

The concept of SD is clinically relevant, particularly in its association with LBP and its prevalence in a clinical setting (Licciardone et al, 2005b) but a clear distinction should be made between clinical evidence and scientific evidence for the concept of SD. SD is more prevalent in subjects with chronic LBP than in subjects without chronic LBP (Snider et al, 2008), and specific OMT is provided on a test-dependent basis for each patient. Patient agreement should also be obtained, and patient values and expectations for the outcome of the OMT should be acknowledged. Although OMT for the treatment of SD associated with LBP is now included in clinical guidelines in the USA, osteopathic practitioners should understand that successful clinical outcomes do not validate this concept. Data from existing clinical, descriptive and physiological studies with strong methodology could only support some of the most common assertions within the osteopathic profession.

As for all other disciplines, osteopathic curricula should rely on the best available evidence, and challenges are arising concerning some osteopathic concepts due to conflicting current evidence (Fryer, 2008). A balance between clinical findings and scientific evidence in osteopathic curricula should therefore be found. Osteopathic practitioners themselves are able to provide critical analysis of their own clinical procedures, and are able to change them according to current scientific evidence (Zegarra-Parodi and Fabre, 2009). For example, OMT training has shifted from expert opinion-based theories (Fryette, 1954) to a more scientific approach (Gibbons and Tehan, 2001; McCarthy, 2001), which includes recent biomechanical studies on spinal coupled movement (Bogduk and Mercer, 2000; Herzog, 2000). Hartmann's minimum leverage techniques concept (Hartmann, 1996) fits with current biomechanical understanding, its main educational objective relying on obtaining pre-manipulative tension with combined leverage on a specific joint and therefore reducing amplitude of the manipulation. Systematically training osteopathic students to find evidence for clinical decisions relative to individual patient needs may be relevant in order to improve their appraisal skills, and use them in a clinical setting once they become professional. This is a long term process. The osteopathic profession has moved from an empirical body of practice to a regulated profession included in different healthcare systems.

Osteopathic medicine is a relatively young profession compared to allopathic medicine, and the lack of scientific studies to support common clinical procedures is currently being addressed, especially in the USA and in the UK; countries where osteopathy was first regulated and where dedicated research institutions now exist: ATSRI and ORC in the USA and the National Council for Osteopathic Research (NCOR) in the UK. The situation is not improved by the fact that there is no regulation or official research facilities in many countries.

5. Conclusion

There is a growing body of clinical evidence to support the use of the concept of SD during osteopathic diagnosis and manipulative treatment for NS-LBP patients. Interpretation of osteopathic palpatory findings is central to the creation of a treatment plan, and the choice of OMT. The concept of SD is also fundamental for osteopathic educators to transmit their experience. This concept is however being challenged owing to the relative lack of scientific evidence, and the current demands from academic and governmental institutions. Successful outcomes in a clinical setting with the use of the SD concept do not equal a validation of this concept. It needs to be re-evaluated in the light of evidence-oriented osteopathy. The SD is currently a clinically descriptive concept rather than one with supporting scientific evidence. The published clinical and experimental data should nevertheless be presented and taught, so that osteopathic practitioners can provide OMT based on the best available levels of evidence.

6. Author contribution statement

RZP designed and planned the book chapter. All authors were involved in data collection and analysis. RZP and JDR wrote the first draft of the manuscript. All authors edited and approved the final version of the manuscript.

7. Acknowledgement

The authors would like to thank Tom Draper-Rodi for English language proofreading of the manuscript.

8. References

Allan, N. Louisa Burns, D.O. J Can Chiropr Assoc 1986;30(2):103-105.

Andersson, G.B.J., Lucente, T., Davis, A.M., Kappler, R.E., Lipton, J.A., & Leurgans, S. A comparison of osteopathic spinal manipulation with standard care for patients with low back pain. N Engl J Med 1999;341:1426-31.

Andrew Taylor Still University (ATSU) Website. Evidence Based Medicine. Available at: http://www.atsu.edu/ebm/step4/index_files/frame.htm. Accessed October 19, 2011.

Authorized Osteopathic Thesaurus. 2009. American Association of Colleges of Osteopathic Medicine Web site. Available at: http://www.aacom.org/resources/bookstore/thesaurus. Accessed October 19, 2011.

American Academy of Osteopathy Website. Outpatient Osteopathic SOAP Note Form Series and Usage Guide. 2nd ed. Indianapolis, Ind: American Academy of Osteopathy; 2002. Available at: http://www.academyofosteopathy.org/files/SOAP_NoteUsageGuide.pdf. Accessed October 19, 2011.

Benchmarks for Training in Osteopathy. 2010. World Health Organization (WHO) Website. Available at: http://whqlibdoc.who.int/publications/2010/9789241599665_eng.pdf . Accessed October 19, 2011.

Bogduk, N., & Mercer, S. Biomechanics of the cervical spine. I: Normal kinematics. Clin Biomech 2000;15(9):633-648.

Bossuyt, P.M., Reitsma, J.B., Bruns, D.E., Gatsonis, C.A., Glasziou, P.P., Irwig, L.M., et al. The STARD statement for reporting studies of diagnostic accuracy: explanation and elaboration. Ann Intern Med 2003;138:W1-12.

Bronfort, G., Haas, M., Evans, R., Leininger, B., & Triano, J. Effectiveness of manual therapies: the UK evidence report. Chiropractic & Osteopathy 2010;18:3.

Brunse, M.H., Stochkendahl, M.J., Vach, W., Kongsted, A., Poulsen, E., Hartvigsen, J., et al. Examination of musculoskeletal chest pain - an inter-observer reliability study. Man Ther 2010;15(2):167-172.

Burns, L. Pathogenesis of visceral disease following vertebral lesions, Chicago: The American Osteopathic Association; 1948.

Carey, T.S., Motyka, T.M., Garrett, J.M., & Keller, R.B. Do osteopathic physicians differ in patient interaction from allopathic physicians ? An empirically derived approach. J Am Osteopath Assoc 2003;103(7):313-318;347-348.

Carnes, D., Mars, T.S., Mullinger, B., Froud, R., & Underwood, M. Adverse events and manual therapy: a systematic review. Man Ther 2010;15(4):355-63.

Degenhardt, B.F., Snider, K.T., Snider, E.J., & Johnson, J.C. Interobserver reliability of osteopathic palpatory diagnostic tests of the lumbar spine: improvements from consensus training. J Am Osteopath Assoc 2005;105:465-473.

Degenhardt, B.F., Darmani, N.A., Johnson, J.C., Towns, L.C., Rhodes, D.C., Trinh, C., Mc Clanahan, B., & Di Marzo, V. Role of osteopathic manipulative treatment in altering pain biomarkers: a pilot study. J Am Osteopath Assoc 2007;107(9):387-400.

Degendardt, B.F. New horizons for research and education in osteopathic manipulative medicine. J Am Osteopath Assoc 2009;109(2):76-78.

Degenhardt, B.F., Johnson, J.C., Snider, K.T., & Snider, E.J. Maintenance and improvement of interobserver reliability of osteopathic palpatory tests over a 4-month period. J Am Osteopath Assoc 2010;110(10):579-86.

Denslow, J.S. The Collected Works of JS Denslow, 1993 Year Book, Indiana: American Academy of Osteopathy; 1993.

Deyo, R.A., & Phillips, W.R.: Low back pain: A primary care challenge. Spine 1996, 21:2826-32.

European Federation of Osteopaths (EFO) Website. The Scope of Osteopathic Practice in Europe. 2010. Available at:
http://www.efo.eu/fc.pdf. Accessed October 19, 2011.

Evans, D.W. Mechanisms and effects of spinal high-velocity, low-amplitude thrust manipulation: previous theories. J Manipulative Physiol Ther 2002;25(4):251-262.

Feinstein, A.R. Clinimetrics. New Haven: Yale University Press; 1987.

Fryette, H. Principles of osteopathic technique. Colorado Springs: The Academy of Applied Osteopathy 1954.

Fryer, G. Somatic Dysfunction: updating the concept. Australian Journal of Osteopathy. 1999;10(2):14-19.

Fryer, G. Intervertebral dysfunction: a discussion of the manipulable spinal lesion. J Ost Med 2003;6(2):64-73.

Fryer, G., Morris, T., & Gibbons, P. Paraspinal muscles and Intervertebral dysfunction: Part One. J Manipulative Physiol Ther. 2004a;27:267-74.

Fryer, G., Morris, T., & Gibbons, P. Paraspinal muscles and Intervertebral dysfunction: Part Two. J Manipulative Physiol Ther 2004b;27:348-57.

Fryer, G., Morris, T., & Gibbons, P. The relation between thoracic paraspinal tissues and pressure sensitivity measured by a digital algometer. J Ost Med 2004c;7(2):64-69.

Fryer, G., Morris, T., Gibbons, P., & Briggs, A. The electromyographic activity of thoracic paraspinal muscles identified as abnormal with palpation. Int J Ost Med 2006;9:27-46.

Fryer, G. Teaching critical thinking in osteopathy - Integrating craft knowledge and evidence-informed approaches. Int J Ost Med 2008;11(2):56-61.

Fryer, G., Bird, M., Morris, B., Fossum, C., & Johnson, J.C. Resting Electromyographic Activity of Deep Thoracic Transversospinalis Muscles Identified as Abnormal With Palpation. J Am Osteopath Assoc 2010a;110(2):61-68.

Fryer, G., Johnson, J.C., & Fossum, C. The use of spinal and sacroiliac joint procedures within the British osteopathic profession. Part 1: Assessment. Int J Ost Med 2010b;13:143-151.

Gibbons, P., & Tehan, P. Patient positioning and spinal locking for lumbar spine rotation manipulation. Man Ther 2001;6(3):130-138.

Hartman, L. Handbook of osteopathic technique. 3rd Edition. Cheltenham: Nelson Thornes Ltd, 1996.

Henderson, A.T., Fischer, J.F., Blair, J., Shea, C., Shan Li, T., & Groves Bridges, K. Effects of Rib raising on the autonomic nervous system: a pilot study using noninvasive biomarkers. J Am Osteopath Assoc 2010;110(6):324-330.

Henley, C.E., Ivins, D., Mills, M., Wen, F.K., & Benjamin, B.A. Osteopathic manipulative treatment and its relationship to autonomic nervous system activity as demonstrated by heart rate variability: a repeated measures study. Osteopathic Medicine and Primary Care 2008;2(7):1-8.

Herzog, W. Clinical biomechanics of spinal manipulation. Philadelphia: Churchill Livingstone, 2000.

Howell, J.N., & Willard, F. Nociception: New Understandings and Their Possible Relation to Somatic Dysfunction and Its Treatment. Ohio Research and Clinical Review 2005;15.

Hoy, D., Brooks, P., Blyth, F., & Buchbinder, R. The epidemiology of low back pain. Best Pract Res Clin Rheumatol 2010;24(6):769-81.

International Classification of Diseases. 2009. World Health Organization Website. Available at: http://apps.who.int/classifications/apps/icd/icd10online/. Accessed October 19, 2011.

Jaeschke, R., Singer, J., & Guyatt, G.H. Measurement of health status. Ascertaining the minimal clinically important difference. Control Clin Trials 1989;10(4):407-15.

Johnson, S.M., & Kurtz, M.E. Osteopathic Manipulative Treatment Techniques Preferred by Contemporary Osteopathic Physicians. J Am Osteopath Assoc 2003;103(5): 219-224.

Johsua, S., & Dupin, J.J. Initiation à la didactique des sciences et des mathématiques; Paris: Presses Universitaires de France, 1993.

Korr, I. The neural basis of the osteopathic lesion. J Am Osteopath Assoc 1947;47:191.

Korr, I. The Collected Papers of Irvin Korr, Indiana: American Academy of Osteopathy; 1979

Korr, I. The Collected Papers of Irvin Korr Vol 2, Indiana: American Academy of Osteopathy; 1997

Kuchera, M.L. Osteopathic manipulative medicine considerations in patients with chronic pain. J Am Osteopath Assoc 2005;105(9 Suppl 4):S29-36.

Kuchera, M.L. Applying Osteopathic Principles to Formulate Treatment for patients with Chronic Pain. J Am Osteopath Assoc 2007;107(6):26-38.

Langevin, H.M. et al. Ultrasound evidence of altered lumbar connective tissue structure in human subjects with chronic low back pain. BMC Musculoskelet Disord. 2009 Dec 3;10:151.

Lederman, E. The science and practice of manual therapy. 2nd edition. Oxford: Churcill Livingstone;2005.

Lee, P.R. Interface: Mechanisms of spirit in osteopathy. Oregon: Stillness Press; 2005.

Leigh, J. The decline & fall of osteopathic medicine. British Osteopathic Journal 1994;13:24-26.

Licciardone, J.C., Stoll, S.T., Fulda, K.G., Russo, D.P., Siu, J., Winn, W., & Swift, J. Osteopathic manipulative treatment for chronic low back pain. A randomized controlled trial. Spine 2003;28:1355-62.

Licciardone, J.C., Brimhall, A.K., & King, L.N. Osteopathic manipulative treatment for low back pain: a systematic review and meta-analysis of randomized controlled trials. BMC musculoskeletal disorders 2005a;6:43.

Licciardone, J.C., Nelson, K.E., Glonek, T., Sleszynski, S.L., & des Anges Cruser. Osteopathic manipulative treatment of somatic dysfunction among patients in the family practice clinic setting: a retrospective analysis. J Am Osteopath Assoc 2005b;105(12):537-44.

Littlejohn, J.M. The theory of the treatment of the spine. The Journal of the Science of Osteopathy 1903 ; 3(6) :258-277.

Lucas, N., & Bogduk, N. Diagnostic reliability in osteopathic medicine. Int J Ost Med 2011;14:43-47.

Manchikanti, L. Epidemiology of low back pain. Pain physician 2000;3(2):167-92.

McCarthy, C.J. Spinal manipulative thrust technique using combined movement theory. Man Ther 2001;6(4):197-204.

Nachemson, A.L. Newest knowledge of low back pain. A critical look. Clin Orthop Relat Res 1992;279:8-20.

NGC-7504. American Osteopathic Association guidelines for osteopathic manipulative treatment (OMT) for patients with low back pain. 2009. National Guidelines Clearinghouse (NGC) Web Site. Available at: http://www.guideline.gov/summary/summary.aspx?view_id=1&doc_id=15271 . Accessed October 19, 2011.

NGC-7704. Guideline for the evidence-informed primary care management of low back pain. 2009. National Guidelines Clearinghouse (NGC) Website. NGC -7704. Available at: http://www.guideline.gov/content.aspx?id=15668&search=low+back+pain. Accessed October 19, 2011.

Pain, Clinical Updates: Low Back Pain. 2010. International Association for the Study of Pain Web Site. Avalaible at: http://www.iasp-pain.org/AM/TemplateRedirect.cfm?template=/CM/ContentDisplay.cfm&ContentID=11730. Accessed October 19, 2011.

Penney, J.N. The biopsychosocial model of pain and contemporary osteopathic practice. International Journal of Osteopathic Medicine 2010;13:42-47

Pickar, J.G. Neurophysiological effects of spinal manipulation. Spine J 2002;2(5): 357-371.

Pincus, T., Vogel, S., Savage, R., & Newman, S. Patient's satisfaction with osteopathic an general practice management of low-back pain in the same surgery. Compl Ther Med 2000;8(3):180-186.

Potter, L., McCarthy, C., & Oldham, J. Physiological effects of spinal manipulation: a review of proposed theories. Phys Ther Rev 2005;10(3):163-170.

Rajendran, D., Mullinger, B., Fossum, C., Collins, P., & Froud, R. Monitoring self-reported adverse events: a prospective, pilot study in a UK osteopathic teaching clinic. Int J Ost Med 2009;12:49-55.

Rogers, F.J., D'Alonzo, G.E. Jr, Glover, J.C., Korr, I.M., Osborn, G.G., Patterson, M.M., & Seffinger, M.A. Proposed tenets of osteopathic medicine and principles for patient care. J Am Osteopath Assoc 2002;102(2):63-5.

Rubinstein, S.M., Van Middelkoop, M., Assendelft, W.J., de Boer, M.R., & van Tulder, M.W. Spinal Manipulative Therapy for Chronic Low-Back Pain: An Update of a Cochrane Review. Spine 2011;36(13):E825-E838.

Rumney, I.C. The relevance of somatic dysfunction. J Am Osteopath Assoc 1975;74(8):723-5.

Sackett, D.L., William, M.C., Rosenberg, W.M.C., Muir Gray, J.A., Haynes, R.B., & Scott Richardson, W. Evidence based medicine: what it is and what it isn't. BMJ 1996;312:71-72.

Seffinger, M.A., Najm, W.I., Mishra, S.I., Adams, A., Vivian, M., Dickerson, V.M., Murphy, L.S., & Reinsch, S. Reliability of Spinal Palpation for Diagnosis of Back and Neck Pain. Spine 2004;29(19):413-425.

Sherman, K.J., Cherkin, D.C., Connelly, M.T., Erro, J., Savetsky, J.B., Davis, R.B., & Eisenberg, D.M. Complementary and alternative medical therapies for chronic low back pain: What treatments are patients willing to try? BMC Complementary and Alternative Medicine 2004;4:9.

Skyba, D.A., Radhakrishnan, R., Rohlwingb, J.J., Wright, A., & Sluka, K.A. Joint manipulation reduces hyperalgesia by activation of monoamine receptors but not opioid or GABA receptors in the spinal cord. Pain 2003;106 :159-168.

Sleszynski, S.L., Gloneck, T., & Kuchera, W.A. Standardized medical record: a new outpatient osteopathic SOAP note form: validation of a standardized office form against physician's progress notes. J Am Osteopath Assoc 1999;10:516-29.

Sleszynski, S.L., & Glonek, T. Outpatient Osteopathic SOAP Note Form: Preliminary Results in Osteopathic Outcomes-Based Research. J Am Osteopath Assoc 2005;4:181-205.

Sloan, T.J., & Walsh, D.A. Explanatory and Diagnostic Labels and Perceived Prognosis in Chronic Low Back Pain. Spine 2010;35:E1120-5

Snider, K.T., Johnson, J.C., Snider, E.J., & Degenhardt, B.F. Increased incidence and severity of somatic dysfunction in subjects with chronic low back pain. J Am Osteopath Assoc 2008;108(8):372-8.

Snider, K.T., Johnson, J.C., Degenhardt, B.F., & Snider, E.J. Low back pain, somatic dysfunction, and segmental bone mineral density T-score variation in the lumbar spine. J Am Osteopath Assoc 2011;111(2):89-96.

Sterling, M., Jull, G., & Wright, A. Cervical mobilisation: concurrent effects on pain, sympathetic nervous system activity and motor activity. Man Ther 2001;6(2):72-81.

Stochkendahl, M.J., Christensen, H.W. et al. Manual examination of the spine: a systematic critical literature review of reproducibility. J Manipulative Physiol Ther 2006;29(6):475-485.

Sun, C., Desai, G.J., Pucci, D.S., & Jew, S. Musculoskeletal disorders: do the osteopathic medical profession demonstrates its unique and distinctive characteristics? J Am Osteopath Assoc 2004;104(4):149-155.

Standard 2000: Standard of proficiency March 1999. General Osteopathic Council (GOsC) Website. Available at: http://www.osteopathy.org.uk/uploads/standard_2000.pdf. Accessed October 19, 2011.

Sturmberg, J.P., & Martin, C.M. Knowing in Medicine. J Eval Clin Pract 2008;14:767-770.

Triano, J.J. Biomechanics of spinal manipulative therapy. The Spine Journal 2001;1:121-130.

Van Buskirk, R.L. Nociceptive reflexes and the somatic dysfunction: a model. J Am Osteopath Assoc 1990;90(9):792-4, 797-809.

Van Dieën, J.H., Cholewicki, J., & Radebold, A. Trunk muscle recruitment patterns in patient with low back pain enhance the stability of the lumbar spine. Spine 2003; 28(8):834-841.

Vogel, S. Adverse events and treatment reactions in osteopathy. Int J Ost Med 2010;13:83-84.

Waddell, G. The Back Pain Revolution Edinburgh: Churchill Livingstone;2004.

Zegarra-Parodi, R., & Fabre, L. Critical analysis of teaching spinal manipulation techniques based on the "Fryette laws". Kinesither Rev 2009;(96):44-47.

Zegarra-Parodi, R. Osteopathy and physical therapy - a gap bridging between two professions. J Phys Ther 2010;1:42-44.